Modern Developments in Livestock Health and Production

Modern Developments *in* Livestock Health and Production

Dr. Dhirendra Kumar
Dr. Vikas Mahajan

SSPH

SATISH SERIAL PUBLISHING HOUSE
403, Express Tower, Commercial Complex
Azadpur, Delhi-110033 (India)
Phone : 011-27672852, Fax : 91-11-27672046
e-mail : info@satishserial.com, hkjain1975@yahoo.com
Website : www.satishserial.com

Published by :

SATISH SERIAL PUBLISHING HOUSE

403, Express Tower, Commercial Complex, Azadpur, Delhi-110033 (INDIA)
Phone : 011-27672852 Fax : 91-11-27672046
E-mail : info@satishserial.com, hkjain1975@yahoo.com

ISBN 978-93-88020-13-8

Composed, Designed & Printed in India

About the Authors

Dr. Dhirendra Kumar is presently working as Assistant Professor of Animal Genetics & Breeding at Sher-e-Kashmir University of Agricultural Sciences and Technology of Jammu (SKUAST-J), R.S.Pura, Jammu (J&K). Dr. Dhirendra is a recipient of Best Ph.D Thesis award, Appreciation Award (2), Distinguished Scientist Award, Excellence in Teaching Award, Young Scientist Award (2) and Life Science Leadership Award. He has also served as Organizing Secretary of International Conference (1), Joint Organizing Secretary of International Conference (1) and Co-Organizing Secretary of National Conference/Symposium (2). Presently he is the Principal Investigator of Network Project of NBAGR-ICAR on Characterization of Poonchi Chicken. He also acted as a Co-Principal Investigator under Network Projects of ICAR on "Characterization of Sheep and Goat". He was the co-project leader of the project "Capacity building /Training of Women Self Help Group members from Umeed as Community Paravets". He has published more than 40 research and review articles in reputed national and international scientific journals. He has edited three books. He has also contributed in scientific fields by means of popular articles, conference proceeding papers, short communications, chapters in books, manuals, edited publications, etc.

Dr. Vikas Mahajan is presently working as Assistant Professor (Ph.D in Animal Genetics & Breeding), Division of Instructional; Livestock Farm Complex, Faculty of Veterinary Sciences and Animal Husbandry, Sher-e-Kashmir University of Agricultural Sciences and Technology of Jammu (SKUAST-J), R.S.Pura, Jammu (J&K). Professional experience more than three years with a wide variety of publication, which includes research papers (23), books (05), manual (02). He has edited two books. He has also contributed in scientific fields by means of popular articles, conference proceeding papers, short communications, chapters in books, manuals, edited publications, etc. He is also reviewer of different National and International Journals.

Preface

The livestock sector is highly vibrant worldwide. In developing country like India, we are budding in response to fast increasing demand for livestock products to nourish the population in a sustainable manner. There are 115 million operational holdings in the country and about 80% of them are marginal and small farmers. To fulfill the basic needs of household including food (cereal, pulses, oilseeds, milk, fruit, honey, meat, etc.), feed, fodder, fiber, etc. warrant an attention about Integrated Farming System (IFS). The production will be affected by struggling for natural resources like land, water and feed. Further, there will be a need for securing the environment while achieving higher production goals by functional control in green house gases. Modern issues like epigenetics impact on livestock nutrition, livestock based integrated farming systems, global warming mitigation through improved livestock management, exogenous fibrolytic enzymes as feed additive and probiotics for better livestock performance.

Improvement or increase in livestock production can be achieved by studying nutritional epigenetics in livestock and modulating the same leading to sustainable food production for human well-being. Livestock production is likely to be affected greatly by environmental factors. Global warming is an international issue mainly due to methane emission, as it appears to be the major cause for global warming. During the process of digestion as a product of enteric fermentation, ruminant serves as a potential source of methane production. Probiotics may improve growth, feed intake, digestibility, ruminal microflora and increase the ruminal fermentation with improvement in rumen pH. Probiotics in the diet will improve the physiological health status of animals. Developments in animal nutrition and health will help to maintain potential production and further increases the efficiency.

The chapters are invited from the various scholars, researchers and academicians throughout the country. We are highly thankful to all the resource persons for their valuable contribution in this book.

The views expressed in this book are solemnly those of the authors. Despite the careful efforts have been made in compilation of present publication, if any error, may kindly be pardoned and brought to the notice for further improvement. We hope the present publication will be useful to the scholars, researchers, policy-makers and academicians in the field of livestock.

Happy Reading

Editors

Contents

1

Epigenetics and Its Impact on Livestock Nutrition

Farukh Mehraj*, Haidar Ali Ahmed*, Yasir Afzal Beigh, Humaira Ashraf and Nazam Khan

* Division of Animal Nutrition, Faculty of Veterinary Sciences and Animal Husbandry, Sher-e-Kashmir University of Agricultural Sciences & Technology of Kashmir, Shuhama, Alusteng, Srinagar-190006 (J&K)

Improvement in animal productivity has been achieved over the years through careful breeding and selection programs. But it is well understood that there exists a substantial gene and environment interaction when considering phenotypic variation. In 1942, Conrad Waddington introduced the term 'epigenetics', meaning outside conventional genetics, to describe events that could not be explained by conventional genetic principles. Epigenetic mechanisms confer heritable, but potentially reversible, states of gene activity that are imposed by the structure of chromatin or covalent modifications of Deoxyribonueleic acid (DNA) and histones. It includes DNA methylation, histone modification, chromatin structure and non-coding RNAs (Cedar and Bergman, 2011). The epigenetic mechanisms have been the focus of some excellent recent reviews (Ibeagha-Awemu and Zhao, 2015; Triantaphyllopoulos *et al.,* 2016). By modifying the chromatin structure, genes are either activated or inactivated depending on the type of epigenetic modification which in turn depends on the environmental stimuli received. This leads to formation of a complete and fully developed individual with hundreds of cell variants having same genotype but different phenotype starting from a single cell zygote. Epigenetics, thus, is a change in phenotype without a change in genotype. Epigenetic factors respond to external or internal environmental cues such as nutrition, pathogens, and climate. Among these, nutrition is one of the most important environmental signals affecting phenotype (Triantaphyllopoulos *et al.,* 2016). Both nutrient quality and quantity play an important role in determining the epigenome of cell.

There is an interaction of specific nutrients with the genetic code possessed by all nucleated cells, which may cause nutritional modulation of the genetic expression for health or disease. The nutrients ingested interact with the genetic code of cells in addition to supporting their metabolism and may result in modulation of the gene expression resulting in health or disease. The impact of nutrition on epigenetics of host and ultimately on the phenotype of host is best demonstrated by honeybee model. The caste system in honey bees is due to the epigenetics (Kucharski *et al.*, 2008). Honeybees grow to be either queens or workers depending on whether they are fed royal jelly or beebread. The different honeybee phenotypes have been suggested to occur through epigenetic changes in DNA methylation patterns induced by the different types of honey. The bee that is fed royal jelly in large quantities and over extended periods turns out to be queen and those that are not fed royal jelly turn into workers. Royal jelly contains major royal jelly proteins and these have been seen to activate genes responsible for reproductive system maturation (Maleszka, 2008). Thus, the bee turns into a fertile queen, whereas others remain infertile. Also, royal jelly contains phenyl butyrate that inhibits histone deacetylases preventing the inactivation of genes needed for the development and maturation of reproductive tract (Lyko *et al.*, 2010). Now, epigenetic marks in brain are also been reported to be affected by the royal jelly explaining the difference in behaviour reported in queen and other females (Chittka and Niven, 2009).

Impact of Epigenetics on the Performance of Livestock

Nutritional epigenetics involves the study of epigenetic mechanisms related to gene-diet interactions (Park *et al.*, 2012). It studies the interaction between nutrition and epigenetics, including the impact of supplementation or biological deficiency of macronutrients, as well as specific micronutrients and secondary plant metabolites on epigenome (Anderson *et al.*, 2012; Murdoch *et al.*, 2016). The main focus of nutritional epigenetics has been on the specific precursors, substrates and enzymes required in the folate cycle, the methionine cycle, and histone methylation, as these relationships are the most direct. Dietary supplementation with folate, choline, or betaine appears to increase DNA methylation because these nutrients are methyl group donors (Anderson *et al.*, 2012; Crider *et al.*, 2012). Also, supplementation with other B vitamins, like B_2, B_6, and B_{12} appear to increase DNA methylation because of their role as co-factors in the methylation process (Powers, 2003; Craig, 2004). Folic acid and betaine have been shown to influence the function of enzymes that participate in the methylation process (VandenVeyver, 2002). Folic acid and betaine undergo a series of chemical reactions resulting in production of methionine (Anderson *et al.,* 2012). Subsequently, methionine is converted to S-adenosyl methionine (SAM), which donates methyl groups to DNA methyl transferases (DNMTs). These DNMTs then covalently attach the methyl groups to the position five of a cytosine base. This suggests that DNA methylation efficiency could be affected by animal nutrition as factors involved in the biochemical pathway that converts nutrients into SAM. When methyl donors, such as folate or betaine are restricted from diet the observation of hypomethylation is generally anticipated. Nutraceuticals and natural foods, such as ω–3 fatty acids, antioxidants, essential and nonessential amino acids, vitamins and minerals, are important for enzyme function and as such suppress the expression of harmful genes. These nutrients are methyl group donors, that is added to the DNA via folate and methionine pathways resulting in DNA methylation. DNA methylation inactivates gene expression leading to well-being of animal. The influence of diet on host genome is well-recognized and a number of studies have conducted in them (Kaati *et al.,* 2007; Waterland *et al.,* 2010; Hossein-nezhad *et al.,* 2013). The effects of different nutrients in humans are presented in table 1. In cattle, dietary supplementation with a rumen protected B-vitamin complex including folate led to increased conception rate at first service suggesting a link between methylation and conception rate in cows (Juchem et al., 2012). Other studies with betaine and other methyl donors are presented in table 2. Not only the methyl donors, imbalanced nutrition also changes the epigenome of cells leading to diseased states in animals. Cows fed a diet rich in unsaturated fatty acids affected the milk fat synthesis and led to differentially regulated profile of (micro RNAs) miRNAs with higher number of miRNAs in subcutaneous and visceral adipose tissues (Romao *et al.,* 2012; Li *et al.,* 2013; 2014). Mineral supplementation has also been shown to impact the health of animal by modulating the epigenome of the cells. The antineoplastic, anti-inflammatory and other effects of minerals are reported to occur via the epigenetic mechanisms (Barrera *et al.,* 2012; Li *et al.,* 2015). Also, ruminants fed high concentrate diets due to a seasonal or regional lack of quality forage material has been seen to lead to acidosis and it accounts for significant economic losses to the livestock industry. Dong and his co-workers reported that in sub-acute ruminal acidosis (SARA), there is accumulation of endotoxin (lipopolysac charide, LPS) in rumen which is then absorbed and leads to inflammatory response in the body including mammary gland. They have reported change in epigenetic marks in the mammary gland due to this LPS implying an indirect impact on nutrition on epigenome in addition to the direct ones already mentioned (Dong *et al.*, 2014). Restricting feeding of pregnant sows lead to reduction of connective tissue and ultimately growth in piglets (Nebendahl *et al.*, 2016).

Table 1: Effects of epigenetic modifications by nutrients in humans

Nutrient	Effect
Refined carbohydrates (sugar and refined starches)	Adverse
Trans fatty acids	Adverse
Excess of saturated fat	Adverse
Excess of linoleic acid	Adverse
ω–3 fatty acids	Beneficial
Monounsaturated fatty acids	Beneficial
Calcium, magnesium, potassium, iron	Beneficial
Zinc, copper, selenium, chromium, manganese, molybdenum, cobalt	Beneficial
Co-enzyme Q10, L-carnitine	Beneficial
Lead, mercury, arsenic, cadmium, fluoride	Adverse
Excess of iron	Adverse
Vitamin A, E, C, D, K and β-carotene and flavonoids	Beneficial
Pyridoxine, thiamin, riboflavin, cyanocobalamin, nicotinic acid, folic acid	Beneficial
Fiber (polysaccharides)	Beneficial
Amino acids: arginine, taurine, cysteine	Beneficial

(Tokunaga *et al.*, 2013)

The epigenome is erased and re-established at fertilization and implantation or blastocyst formation respectively with continuous changes occurring during development. This occurs so that new totipotent cells formed can form the new individual with all its tissues and organs. This erasing and re-establishing period represent critical times or "windows" in which any environmental cue including nutritional changes or disruptions may be perpetuated. Any change during these critical windows of time can directly affect the developing animal and/or the cells that contribute to future generations (Ficz *et al.*, 2011). The agouti coat colour phenotype in mice has been shown to be influenced by maternal diet (Waterland and Jirtle, 2004). Barker *et al.* (1989, 1990 and 1993) reported a link between maternal malnourishment with prevalence of heart disease, hypertension and type 2 diabetes in progeny. Dietary fatty acids may promote establishment of epigenetic marks by stimulating expression of specific genes during critical periods of growth like peroxisome proliferator activated receptor-α (PPAR-α) transcription factor (Waterland and Rached, 2006). Martin and co-workers reported that if the diet of cows is supplemented with protein in last trimester, it led to early conception in first breeding season and overall greater pregnancy rates in offsprings (Martin *et al.*, 2007) and also protein supplement in second trimester to cows led to decreased number of antral follicles in heifers at 2 years of age (Sullivan *et al.*, 2009). Similarly, in pigs, maternal low-protein diet during gestation and lactation led to abnormal homeostasis in the offspring (Cong *et al.*, 2012). Alteration in Insulin-like growth factor (IGF) receptor number and leptin gene transcription in adipose tissue was reported to be altered by the maternal nutrient intake (Micke *et al.*, 2011). In other studies, heifers fed low protein diets (70% of recommended) during first trimester had higher cross-sectional areas of longissimus dorsi and semitendinosus (ST) muscles in mature male progeny, whereas heifers fed high protein diets (240%) had heavier calves (Micke *et al.*, 2010; 2011). The primary energy source fed to dams during pregnancy has been reported to affect the offspring phenotype. Calves from dams fed corn had the lowest marbling score but with greater birth weights (Radunz *et al.*, 2012). Similarly, in sheep, lambs from ewes fed dried corn distillers grains had a greater initial insulin response, dressing percentage, internal fat, lower calculated boneless trimmed retail cuts percentage and increased fetal subcutaneous and peri-renal adipose with higher expression of dephosphorylation, phosphatase activity, and phosphoric ester hydrolase activity genes. Whereas, lambs from corn fed ewes had better myogenesis with decreased expression of genes involved in energetic metabolism, including those implicated in glycolysis and gluconeogenesis, citrate cycle, and valine, leucine and isoleucine degradation (Peñagaricano *et al.*, 2014). So, utmost importance must be given to diet of pregnant animals particularly in the critical periods as phenotypic traits are heavily impacted in this period.

Milk from domestic animals form a critical component of the human diet. The composition of milk depends on the nutrition of the animal and there are about 245 miRNAs in cow milk (Chen *et al.*, 2010; Izumi *et al.*, 2012). These are absorbed by the humans and have been showed to affect the transcriptome of human peripheral blood mononuclear cells (PBMCs), mouse liver cells. One of the miRNAs, miR-200c, has been shown to decrease cancer risk by targeting the transcription factor ZEB1 (Baier *et al.*, 2014). Further research needs to be done to explore effects of these miRNAs on offspring as well as human health. Also, the miRNA composition can be changed via nutrition. This may provide an opportunity to promote production of designer milk with prominent health benefits.

Epigenetic marks are inheritable

Nutrition not only affects epigenome of the consumer, it also impacts progeny performance. Environmentally induced changes in the epigenome have been recorded in genomic DNA methylation patterns for up to three generations (Daxinger *et al.*, 2010). In case of livestock, transmittance of epigenetic patterns was first reported in pigs for iodotyrosine deiodinase gene (Braunschweig *et al.*, 2012). Similarly, diet of pregnant ewes has been reported to affect the weight of their grand daughters (Nijland *et al.*, 2008). Hence, improvement in livestock can be achieved by modulating epigenome of current generation by improved management, specific nutritional regimes to obtain desired phenotypes, design of epigenetic therapies and correction/introduction of epigenome variation by epigenome editing technologies and also by studying the inheritance of epigenetic marks. With the improvement in genetic composition, this epigenetic inheritance could play a driving role in productivity improvement, especially in the animals with shorter generation intervals and that produce large number of offspring like swine and poultry. Many studies have implicated the impact of plane of nutrition of the dam on offspring phenotype. Further research is needed in this area of epigenetics and how dam nutrition affects both the qualitative and quantitative traits of offspring and the future generations.

Table 2: Examples of nutritional mediated alterations of epigenetics in livestock.

Dietary change	Epigenetic effects	Outcome	Species	Reference
Dietary supplementation of Vitamin B Vitamin B_{12},	DNA methylation (axin fused allele affected)	Healthy puppies not prone to diabetes	Mice	Waterland *et al.*, 2006
Folate and methionine eficient	Hypomethylation in methyl-deficient diet	Male progeny had an estimated 25% greater body fat, higher blood pressure, insulin resistance	Sheep	Sinclair *et al.*, 2007
Methylating micronutrients	IYD gene differentially methylated between groups of pigs with extreme obesity related phenotypes	Had more muscle mass at shoulders were leaner	Pigs	Braunschweig *et al.*, 2012
Maternal protein insufficiency	Hypomethylationinpro-opiomelanocortin (POMC) and glucocorticoid receptor(GR) in the sheep brain	Changes in fetal hypothalamic pathways regulating metabolism. Obesity and diabetes	Sheep	Begum *et al.*, 2012
Selenium	Inhibits DNMT1 (induction of GSTP1, APC and CSR1 gene)	Antineoplastic effect	Rats	Barrera *et al.*, 2012
Folic acid supplementation	Hypermethylation in intrauterine growth restriction (IUGR) piglets	Normal birth weight restored	Pigs	Jing-boet *al.*, 2013
Unsaturated fatty acids rich diet	Histone modification	Milk fat synthesis affected	Cow	Li et *al.*, 2013
Unsaturated fatty acids rich diet	Unknown	Higher number of miRNAs in subcutaneous and visceral adipose tissues differentially	Cow	Romaoet *al.*, 2012 Li *et al.*, 2014

		regulated profile of miRNAs		
High concentrate diets	Methylation of the SCD gene (associated with milk fat synthesis) Methylation of STAT5A A involved in protein synthesis	Reduce milk fat synthesis Enhanced protein synthesis	Cows	Dong *et al.*, 2014
Betaine supplementation	PEPCK1 gene hypomethylated and enriched for H3K27 me3. PEPCK2 and FBP1 genes hypermethylated and enriched for H3K4me3	More hepatic gluconeogenic capability	Neonatal Piglets	Cai *et al.*, 2014
Betaine supplementation	Increased global measures of DNA methylation	Improved animal performance. More efficient use of dietary protein. Alterations in the distribution pattern of protein and fat in the body.	Chicks	Hu *et al.*, 2015
High fat diet	Epigenetic regulation of the fatty acid desaturase gene (Fads2)	Changes in hepatic polyunsaturated fatty acid (PUFA) status in offspring	Rats	Mennitti *et al.*, 2015
Zinc supplementation	Hypomethylation and increased expression of gene A20	Reduced intestinal inflammation	Hens	Li *et al.*, 2015
Variable zinc levels	Hypermethylation in regulatory regions of gene ZIP4	Maintaining Zn homeostasis	Piglets	Karweina *et al.*, 2015
Restrictive feeding	Increased global measures of H3K9 acetylation and reduction in H3K9 me3 in IUGR pigs subjected to restrictive feeding	Reduction of connective tissue and growth retardation ion piglets	Pigs	Nebendahlet *al.*, 2016

Summary

Improvement or increase in livestock production can be achieved by studying nutritional epigenetics in livestock and modulating the same leading to sustainable food production. The effect of nutrition to the epigenome of animal is in its infancy though various studies have already implicated the role of nutrition affecting livestock phenotypic traits. Epigenetic studies will allow for the improvement of current livestock population as well as the future one because of its inheritable nature. Also, different livestock products for human composition can be modified so as to improve the health of humans also. The epigenetic abnormalities in cloned animals can be catered with proper understanding of the field of epigenetics and how nutrition plays a role. With the genome sequence of most of the animals now known, the field of epigenetics is likely to flourish at a tremendous pace.

References

1. Anderson, O.S., Sant, K.E. and Dolinoy, D.C., 2012. Nutrition and epigenetics: an interplay of dietary methyl donors, one-carbon metabolism and DNA methylation. The Journal of nutritional biochemistry, **23**(8): 853-859. doi:10.1016/j.jnutbio.2012.03.003
2. Baier, S.R., Nguyen, C., Xie, F., Wood, J.R. and Zempleni, J., 2014. MicroRNAs are absorbed in biologically meaningful amounts from nutritionally relevant doses of cow milk and affect gene expression in peripheral blood mononuclear cells, HEK-293 kidney cell cultures, and mouse livers. The Journal of nutrition, **144**(10): 1495-1500.
3 Barker, D.J., Bull, A.R., Osmond, C. and Simmonds, S.J., 1990. Fetal and placental size and risk of hypertension in adult life. British Medical Journal, **301**: 259–262.
4. Barker, D.J., Hales, C.N., Fall, C.H., Osmond, C., Phipps, K. and Clark, P.M., 1993. Type 2 (non-insulin-dependent) diabetes mellitus, hypertension and hyperlipidaemia (syndrome X): relation to reduced fetal growth. Diabetologia, **36**: 62–67.
5. Barker, D.J., Winter, P.D., Osmond, C., Margetts, B. and Simmonds, S.J., 1989. Weight in infancy and death from ischaemic heart disease. Lancet, 577–580.
6. Barrera, L.N., Cassidy, A., Johnson, I.T., Bao, Y. and Belshaw, N.J., 2012. Epigenetic and antioxidant effects of dietary isothiocyanates and selenium: potential implications for cancer chemoprevention.

Proceedings of the Nutrition Society, **71**(2): 237-245. doi: 10.1017/S002966511200016X

7. Begum, G., Stevens, A., Smith, E.B., Connor, K., Challis, J.R., Bloomfield, F. and White, A., 2012. Epigenetic changes in fetal hypothalamic energy regulating pathways are associated with maternal undernutrition and twinning. The FASEB Journal, **26**(4): 1694-1703.
8. Braunschweig, M., Jagannathan, V., Gutzwiller, A. and Bee, G. 2012., Investigations on transgenerational epigenetic response down the male line in F2 pigs. PLoS ONE,**7**: e30583. doi: 10.1371/journal.pone.0030583.
9. Cai, D., Jia, Y., Song, H., Sui, S., Lu, J., Jiang, Z. and Zhao, R., 2014. Betaine supplementation in maternal diet modulates the epigenetic regulation of hepatic gluconeogenic genes in neonatal piglets. PloS ONE, **9**(8): e105504.
10. Cedar, H. and Bergman, Y., 2011. Epigenetics of haematopoietic cell development. Nature Reviews Immunology, **11**(7): 478-488.
11. Chen, X., Gao, C., Li, H., Huang, L., Sun, Q., Dong, Y., Tian, C., Gao, S., Dong, H., Guan, D. and Hu, X., 2010. Identification and characterization of microRNAs in raw milk during different periods of lactation, commercial fluid, and powdered milk products. Cell research, **20**(10): 1128-1137.
12. Chittka, L. and Niven, J., 2009. Are Bigger Brains Better? Current Biology, **19**: 995–1008.
13. Cong, R., Jia, Y., Li, R., Ni, Y., Yang, X., Sun, Q., Parvizi, N. and Zhao, R., 2012. Maternal low-protein diet causes epigenetic deregulation of HMGCR and CYP7á1 in the liver of weaning piglets. The Journal of nutritional biochemistry, **23**(12): 1647-1654.
14. Craig, S.A., 2004. Betaine in human nutrition. The American journal of clinical nutrition, **80**(3): 539-549.
15. Crider, K.S., Yang, T.P., Berry, R.J. and Bailey, L.B., 2012. Folate and DNA methylation: a review of molecular mechanisms and the evidence for folate's role. Advances in Nutrition: An International Review Journal, **3**(1): 21-38. doi:10.3945/an.111.000992
16. Daxinger, L. and Whitelaw, E., 2010. Transgenerational epigenetic inheritance: more questions than answers. Genome research, **20**(12): 1623-1628. doi: 10.1101/gr.106138.110
17. Dong, G., Qiu, M., Ao, C., Zhou, J., Wang, X., Zhang, Z. and Yang, Y., 2014. Feeding a high-concentrate corn straw diet induced

epigenetic alterations in the mammary tissue of dairy cows. PLoS ONE, **9**(9): e107659.

18. Ficz, G., Branco, M.R., Seisenberger, S., Santos, F., Krueger, F., Hore, T.A., Marques, C.J., Andrews, S. and Reik, W., 2011. Dynamic regulation of 5-hydroxymethylcytosine in mouse ES cells and during differentiation. Nature, **473**(7347): 398-402. doi:10.1038/nature 10008

19. Hossein-Nezhad, A., Spira, A. and Holick, M.F., 2013. Influence of vitamin D status and vitamin D3 supplementation on genome wide expression of white blood cells: a randomized double-blind clinical trial. PloS one, **8**(3): e58725.

20. Hu, Y., Sun, Q., Li, X., Wang, M., Cai, D., Li, X. and Zhao, R., 2015. In ovo injection of betaine affects hepatic cholesterol metabolism through epigenetic gene regulation in newly hatched chicks. PloS one, **10**(4): e0122643.

21. Ibeagha-Awemu, E.M. and Zhao, X., 2015. Epigenetic marks: regulators of livestock phenotypes and conceivable sources of missing variation in livestock improvement programs. Frontiers in genetics, **6**:302. doi:10.3389/fgene.2015.00302

22. Izumi, H., Kosaka, N., Shimizu, T., Sekine, K., Ochiya, T. and Takase, M., 2012. Bovine milk contains microRNA and messenger RNA that are stable under degradative conditions. Journal of dairy science, **95**(9): 4831-4841.

23. Jingbo, L., Ying, Y., Bing, Y., Xiangbing, M., Zhiqing, H., Guoquan, H., Hong, C. and Daiwen, C., 2013. Folic acid supplementation prevents the changes in hepatic promoter methylation status and gene expression in intrauterine growth retarded piglets during early weaning period. Journal of animal physiology and animal nutrition, **97**(5): 878-886. doi: 10.1111/j.1439-0396.2012.01333.x

24. Juchem, S.O., Robinson, P.H. and Evans, E., 2012. A fat based rumen protection technology post-ruminally delivers a B vitamin complex to impact performance of multiparous Holstein cows. Animal feed science and technology, **174**(1): 68-78. doi: 10.1016 j. anifee dsci. 2012.03.004

25. Kaati, G., Bygren, L.O., Pembrey, M. and Sjöström, M., 2007. Transgenerational response to nutrition, early life circumstances and longevity. European Journal of Human Genetics, **15**(7): 784-790.

26. Karweina, D., Kreuzer-Redmer, S., Müller, U., Franken, T., Pieper, R., Baron, U., Olek, S., Zentek, J. and Brockmann, G.A., 2015. The zinc concentration in the diet and the length of the feeding period

affect the methylation status of the ZIP4 zinc transporter gene in piglets. PloS one, **10**(11): e0143098.

27. Kucharski, R., Maleszka, J., Foret, S. and Maleszka, R., 2008. Nutritional control of reproductive status in honeybees via DNA methylation. Science, **319**(5871): 1827-1830. doi: 10.1126/science.1153069

28. Li, C., Guo, S., Gao, J., Guo, Y., Du, E., Lv, Z. and Zhang, B., 2015. Maternal high-zinc diet attenuates intestinal inflammation by reducing DNA methylation and elevating H3K9 acetylation in the A20 promoter of offspring chicks. The Journal of nutritional biochemistry, **26**(2): 173-183. doi: 10.1016/j.jnutbio.2014.10.005.

29. Li, R., Beaudoin, F., Zhao, X. and Ibeagha-Awemu E. M. 2013. "Possible involvement of epigenetic modifying enzymes in the regulation of nutrient effect on bovine milk fat synthesis," in Proceedings of the CSAS-CMSA 2013 Joint Annual Meeting (Banff Alberta, AB: Banff Park Lodge Resort Hotel and Conference Centre;

30. Li, R., Beaudoin, F., Zhao, X., Lei, C. and Ibeagha-Awemu, E. M. 2014. "MicroRNAs are involved in bovine mammary gland response to dietary supplementation with saower oil," in Proceedings of the 10th World Congress on Genetics Applied to Livestock Production Vancouva, BC, 3.

31. Lyko, F., Foret, S., Kucharski, R., Wolf, S., Falckenhayn, C. and Maleszka, R., 2010. The honey bee epigenomes: differential methylation of brain DNA in queens and workers. PLoS biology, **8**(11): e1000506.

32. Maleszka, R., 2008. Epigenetic integration of environmental and genomic signals in honey bees: the critical interplay of nutritional, brain and reproductive networks. Epigenetics, **3**(4): 188-192.

33. Martin, J.L., Vonnahme, K.A., Adams, D.C., Lardy, G.P. and Funston, R.N., 2007. Effects of dam nutrition on growth and reproductive performance of heifer calves. Journal of Animal Science, **85**(3): 841-847. doi: 10.2527/jas.2006-337

34. Mennitti, L.V., Oliveira, J.L., Morais, C.A., Estadella, D., Oyama, L.M., do Nascimento, C.M.O. and Pisani, L.P., 2015. Type of fatty acids in maternal diets during pregnancy and/or lactation and metabolic consequences of the offspring. The Journal of nutritional biochemistry, **26**(2): 99-111. doi: 10.1016/j.jnutbio.2014.10.001.

35. Micke, G.C., Sullivan, T.M., McMillen, I.C., Gentili, S. and Perry, V.E.A., 2011. Protein intake during gestation affects postnatal bovine

skeletal muscle growth and relative expression of IGF1, IGF1R, IGF2 and IGF2R. Molecular and cellular endocrinology, **332**(1): 234-241. doi: 10.1016/j.mce.2010.10.018

36. Micke, G.C., Sullivan, T.M., Gatford, K.L., Owens, J.A. and Perry, V.E.A., 2010. Nutrient intake in the bovine during early and mid-gestation causes sex-specific changes in progeny plasma IGF-I, liveweight, height and carcass traits. Animal reproduction science, **121**(3): 208-217.
37. Murdoch, B.M., Murdoch, G.K., Greenwood, S. and McKay, S., 2016. Nutritional Influence on Epigenetic Marks and Effect on Livestock Production. Frontiers in genetics, 7.
38. Nebendahl, C., Görs, S., Albrecht, E., Krüger, R., Martens, K., Giller, K., Hammon, H.M., Rimbach, G. and Metges, C.C., 2016. Early postnatal feed restriction reduces liver connective tissue levels and affects H3K9 acetylation state of regulated genes associated with protein metabolism in low birth weight pigs. The Journal of nutritional biochemistry, **29**: 41-55. doi: 10.1016/j.jnutbio.2015.10.017
39. Nijland, M.J., Ford, S.P. and Nathanielsz, P.W., 2008. Prenatal origins of adult disease. Current opinion in obstetrics and gynecology, **20**(2): 132-138. doi: 10.1097GCO.0b013e3282f76753
40. Park, L.K., Friso, S. and Choi, S.W., 2012. Nutritional influences on epigenetics and age-related disease. Proceedings of the nutrition society, **71**(1): 75-83.
41. Peñagaricano, F., Wang, X., Rosa, G.J., Radunz, A.E. and Khatib, H., 2014. Maternal nutrition induces gene expression changes in fetal muscle and adipose tissues in sheep. BMC genomics, **15**(1): 1034.
42. Powers, H.J. 2003. Riboflavin (vitaminB-2) and health. The American journal of clinical nutrition, **77**: 1352-1360.
43. Radunz, A.E., Fluharty, F.L., Relling, A.E., Felix, T.L., Shoup, L.M., Zerby, H.N. and Loerch, S.C., 2012. Prepartum dietary energy source fed to beef cows: II. Effects on progeny postnatal growth, glucose tolerance, and carcass composition. Journal of animal science, **90**(13): 4962-4974.
44. Romao, J. M., Jin, W., He, M., Mcallister, T., and Guan L. L. 2012. Altered microRNA expression in bovine subcutaneous and visceral adipose tissues from cattle under different diet. PLoS ONE, **7**: e40605
45. Sinclair, K.D., Allegrucci, C., Singh, R., Gardner, D.S., Sebastian, S., Bispham, J., Thurston, A., Huntley, J.F., Rees, W.D., Maloney, C.A. and Lea, R.G., 2007. DNA methylation, insulin resistance, and blood

pressure in offspring determined by maternal periconceptional B vitamin and methionine status. Proceedings of the national academy of sciences, **104**(49): 19351-19356. doi:10.1073/pnas.0707258104

46. Sullivan, T.M., Micke, G.C., Greer, R.M., Irving-Rodgers, H.F., Rodgers, R.J. and Perry, V.E.A., 2009. Dietary manipulation of *Bos indicus* × heifers during gestation affects the reproductive development of their heifer calves. Reproduction, fertility and development, **21**(6): 773-784. doi: 10.1071/RD09004
47. Tokunaga, M., Takahashi, T., Singh, R.B., De Meester, F. and Wilson, D.W., 2013. Nutrition and epigenetics. Medical epigenetics, **1**(1): 70-77.
48. Triantaphyllopoulos, K.A., Ikonomopoulos, I., and Bannister, A.J., 2016. Epigenetics and inheritance of phenotype variation in livestock. Epigenetics Chromatin, **9**: 31. doi:10.1186/s13072-016-0081-5
49. Van den Veyver, I.B., 2002. Genetic effects of methylation diets. Annual review of nutrition, **22**(1): 255-282.
50. Waterland, R.A., Dolinoy, D.C., Lin, J.R., Smith, C.A., Shi, X. and Tahiliani, K.G., 2006. Maternal methyl supplements increase offspring DNA methylation at Axin Fused. Genesis, **44**: 401-406. doi: 10.1002/dvg.20230.
51. Waterland, R.A., Kellermayer, R., Laritsky, E., Rayco-Solon, P., Harris, R.A., Travisano, M., Zhang, W., Torskaya, M.S., Zhang, J., Shen, L., Manary, M.J. and Prentice, A.M. 2010. Season of conception in rural Gambia affects DNA methylation at putative human metastable epialleles. PLoS Genetics **6**: e1001252.
52. Waterland, R.A. and Rached, M.T., 2006. Developmental establishment of epigenotype: a role for dietary fatty acids?. Scandinavian Journal of Food and Nutrition, **50**(sup2): 21-26.
53. Waterland, R. A. and Jirtle, R.L. 2004.Early nutrition, epigenetic changes at transposons and imprinted genes, and enhanced susceptibility to adult chronic diseases. Nutrition, **20**: 63-68. doi:10.1016/j.nut.2003.09.011.

□□□

2

Role of Toll like Receptor(s) in Tumor Biology and Pathogen Recognition

Mir Mudasir*, Nawab Nashiruddullah, S. Khandi, Nazam Khan, Dhirendra Kumar, G.A Badroo, Faizan Javid & Raja Waseem Yousuf

* Division of Veterinary Pathology, F.V.Sc & A.H, R.S Pura, SKUAST-J-181102

TLRs belong to the pattern recognition receptors (PRR) family that is designed to sense both self and non-self danger signals (Singh *et al.*, 2012). They play a crucial role in innate immune system, and act as first line of defense against various pathogens (Andersen *et al.*, 2006). TLRs recognize large number of molecular structures which includes lipopeptides, lipopolysaccharides lipoteichoic acids, peptidoglycans, zymogens, mannans, flagellins, viral and bacterial nucleic acids, etc. They cause activation of inflammatory cytokines like the interferons, the interleukins IL2, IL6, IL8, IL12, IL16, and TNF-α (as one of the responses) by initiating signal transduction cascades resulting in to get rid of unwanted organisms, pathogens and transformed self tissues to maintain cellular homeostasis (Pradhan *et al.*, 2012). Based on ligand (pathogen) recognition, TLR signaling can trigger different processes in the cell including apoptosis, opsonization and phagocytosis, induction of reactive oxygen/nitrogen species and activation of the complement pathway (Tipping, 2006). Furthermore, activation of TLRs is also known to activate intracellular signaling pathways resulting in activation of transcription factors including NFκB, MAPK, etc. NF-κB regulates expression of anti-apoptotic genes, cytokines and growth factors [Singh and Pollard, 2015). Till date, eleven different TLRs have been identified in humans (Kawai and Akira, 2006) which play an important role in the initiation of adaptive immune responses (Hoebe *et al.*, 2004). Pathogen (ligand) specific adaptive immunity develops due to activation of antigen presentation, TLR-dependent expression of pro inflammatory cytokines and up regulation of co-stimulatory molecules (Husebye *et al.*, 2006). Moreover, T lymphocytes also express selective TLRs and can be directly activated by their respective ligands (Kabelitz, 2007). TLRs have also been shown to be an important link between innate and adaptive immunity (Husebye *et al.*, 2006). TLR signaling plays an important role in maintenance of cellular homeostasis and influences cell proliferation or apoptosis, cell differentiation, as well as induction of different chemokines, inflammatory cytokines including interleukins and interferons (Kanzler *et al.*, 2007). Both the innate and acquired immune system renders protection to organism from foreign pathogens and altered self-tissues while sustaining immune tolerance to normal self-tissues. TLRs play twin, but contrasting role in tumor biology. They maintain antitumor environment by eliciting activation of antitumor mediators, such as type I interferon (Yoon *et al.*, 2012) .TLRs are even documented to play supportive role for initiation, progression and metastasis of cancer (Alderton, 2012).

Structure and Activation

TLRs are trans membrane proteins which play a critical role in innate and adaptive immune responses by initiating the signal transduction cascades after interaction with specific pathogen associated molecular patterns (PAMP) ligands (Bell *et al.*, 2003). Some types of TLR, such as TLR1, TLR2, TLR4, TLR5, TLR6, and TLR11 are located on the cell surface while TLR3, TLR7, TLR8, and TLR9 are associated with the endosomal/lysosomal compartment. TLRs are expressed on cells of the adaptive immunity (T and B lymphocytes), membranes of dendritic cells, macrophages, natural killer cells, and non-immune cells (epithelial, endothelial cells, and fibroblasts). TLR1 is predominantly distributed in monocytes/macrophages and PMNs. TLR2 can be found on immune cells including neutrophils, macrophages, and dendritic cells, but also on stromal cells throughout the body. Most of the TLRs are expressed at low to undetectable levels in human naive B cells while as expression of TLR9 and TLR10 is highly increased following B-cell receptors (BCR) activation. Memory B cells express several TLRs at constitutively high levels.

TLRs can be activated by various PAMPs. They form non-covalent dimers. All the TLRs forms homodimers except TLR2 which forms heterodimer with either TLR1 or TLR6. The cytoplasmic domains of TLRs are known as Toll/Interleukin-1 receptor (TIR) domains due to their structural homology with interleukin-1 Receptor (IL-1R) signaling domain. An adaptor protein is recruited via TIR domain after the specific ligand activation of the TLR receptor. Specific adaptor proteins include MyD88, Mal (MyD88 adaptor-like)/TIRAP (TIR domain-containing adaptor protein), TRIF (TIR domain-containing adaptor inducing interferon beta), TRAM (Trif related adaptor molecule), and SARM (SAM and ARM containing protein). Binding of adaptor proteins leads to the downstream activation of different transcription factors including MAP kinases (JNK, p38 MAPK) and NF-êB. Activation of My D88-independent pathways occurs via TRIF and TRAF3.

Evolution and Organization of Toll Gene

DNA sequence comparisons of genes encoding Toll-related proteins in Drosophila, reptiles, birds and mammals have revealed that the genes are well conserved and have evolved independently from a common ancestor gene. Drosophila genome contains nine TLR genes encoding Toll and related receptors (dToll1–dToll9), whereas in mice and humans, ten TLR genes have been identified (Rock *et al.*, 1998).

Role of TLR in Innate and Acquired Immunity

TLRs act as a bridge between innate and adaptive immunity through their presence on the dendritic cells and by mediating dendritic cell maturation and activation of pathogen specific T lymphocytes. Dendritic cells (DCs) are the potent Antigeni presenting cells and descend through both myeloid and lymphoid lineages. They express both MHC class II and members of co-stimulatory B7 family (CD80 and CD86). Detection of microbial infection and subsequent activation of inflammatory and antimicrobial innate immune responses depends on specificity of the TLRs for products of microbial origin. TLR ligands are products of either prokaryotic, viral or protozoan metabolism, and TH1 responses are required for protection against pathogens of these classes. TH2 responses, by contrast, are protective against multicellular eukaryotic parasites, such as helminthes (Akira and Takeda, 2005). Immature DCs are mainly located in peripheral tissues particularly at the pathogen-entry sites, where they can detect and capture microbial invaders. These immature DCs express a full set of TLRs which induce DC maturation. Mature DCs migrate to draining lymph nodes where they present pathogen-derived antigens to naive T cells. The pathogen associated molecular pattern (PAMPs) are first detected by TLRs present on the dendritic cells which result in transcription of cytokine genes in the nucleus of DCs cells and leads to production of instructive cytokines (IL 12, IL 18 etc.) and expression of co-stimulatory molecules. Further the pathogens are internalized by DC cells broken down into peptides and display the peptides along with MHC class II molecules on the surface of DC cells. This peptide MHC complex is recognized by naïve T cells and with the help of instructive cytokines produced early in the infection, differentiation of naïve T cells into TH1 cells and TH2 cells mediated by IL12,18 and IL 4 respectively. TH1 cells produce IFN-ã and mediate cellular immunity while as TH2 cells produce IL 4, 5, 10, 13 and promote mainly humoral immunity (Banchereau and Steinman, 1998).

TLRS and Tolerance

Data arising predominantly from human patients and animal models of auto immune diseases indicates that inappropriate triggering of TLR pathways by exogenous and endogenous ligands may cause perpetuation of auto immune reactions and tissue damage. Auto immunity relates to presence of auto reactive immune cell subsets and loss of immunological tolerance. Central tolerance is mediated through mechanism of clonal deletion of auto reactive immune cells (bone marrow and thymus). Peripheral tolerance is another branch of immunological tolerance which take place after B and T cells egress from primary lymphoid organs, the main purpose of which is to ensure that self reactive B and T cells which escaped central tolerance don't cause auto immune diseases (tissues and lymphoid nodes). Loss of tolerance is attributed to certain factors like genetic predisposition, self antigenic load, expression of co-stimulatory molecules during APC maturation and absence of T regulatory function during development of adaptive immune response. TLR molecules and their downstream signaling pathways play a critical role in activating innate and adaptive immune responses. Their specific role in modulating immune response also interferes with the mechanism that maintains tolerance in the host. The continuous activation/ dysregulation of TLR signaling might contribute to pathogenesis of autoimmune diseases like systemic lupus erthyromatosis, rheumatoid arthritis, etc. (Hosseini *et al.*, 2015).

TLR Agonists: Role in Cancer Progression

Local irritation and chronic inflammation promote survival, proliferation and migration of cancer cells and is known to enhance tumor development and progression (Dadi *et al.*, 2016). Various factors that determine the tumor stimulating effect of TLRs are interaction of TLRs with its own ligands induces the activation of the NF-κB transcription factor and results in increase in the production of various pro-inflammatory cytokines (IL-6, MCP-1, MIF, GRO-α, etc.), as well as a number of anti-apoptotic proteins, which facilitates direct or indirect tumor-stimulating effect. Activation of myeloid cells and their progenitors by TLR is apparently the determining factor in the formation of metastasis. A series of independent works have demonstrated that myeloid cells migrating from the bone marrow (in response to endogenous stimulation) into tissues play a key role in the formation of metastasis niches (Dietsch *et al.*, 2015). Since endogenous (versican, fibronectin, etc.) and exogenous (microbial origin) TLR ligands are known to be capable of stimulating myeloid cells and their progenitors and increasing the metastatic potential of the tumor, it is very likely that an interrelationship exists between the TLR-dependent activation of myeloid cells and their subsequent involvement in metastasis. TLR activation can stimulate angiogenesis via angiogenic factors, such as IL-8, vascular endothelial growth factor (VEGF), and matrix metalloproteinases (MMP), as well as enhance the adhesive and invasive activity of tumor cells, in line with the increase in the permeability of blood vessels.

TLR Agonists: Role in Anti Tumor Therapy

Cytotoxic T lymphocytes play a pivotal role in tumor immune surveillance by specifically recognizing and killing tumor cells and maintaining tumor-specific immune memory (Gajewski *et al.*, 2013). However, cancer cells are self-derived and generally poor immunogens; can bypass immuno-surveillance by lack of antigen-specific T cell responses. A variety of mechanisms including the induction of eTregs help the tumors evade the elimination and equilibrium phases of cancer immuno-editing (Dadi *et al.*, 2016). TLR agonists are identified as powerful immune adjuvants for antigen-presenting cells (APC) activation. Activation of APCs through TLRs has been exploited by numerous traditional chemotherapeutic drugs that trigger innate and adaptive immune activation (Gajewski *et al.*, 2013). Bacterial lipoprotein (BLP) has been shown to mediate tumor regression by abolishing eTregs function (Zhang *et al.*, 2011). TLR agonists trigger rapid and co-ordinated modulation of immune response including activation of immune cells (lymphocytes, leukocytes, etc.), production of inflammatory mediators, chemokines, cytokines that leads to the generation of cellular (adaptive) immune responses (Vacchelli *et al.*, 2103). These events hold promising applications for the treatment of inflammation and cancer (Northfelt *et al.*, 2014). Several TLR agonists are currently being investigated for their antitumor efficacy and are currently under different stages of drug development (Vacchelli *et al.*, 2013). However, BCG is the only US-FDA approved TLR agonist as a standalone therapeutic intervention. TLR agonists are increasingly explored for their ability to enhance immune responses against tumors and infectious agents (Gearing, 2007). They have an ability to stimulate APCs resulting in activation of tumor-specific T cell responses (Alderton, 2012). Thus, selective down regulation of eTreg function, coupled with the promotion of cytotoxic T lymphocyte (CTL) activity, may represent an attractive strategy for future cancer immunotherapy (Zhang *et al.*, 2011).

Regulation of TLR Expression

TLR expression is regulated in both a cell type and stimulus-dependent fashion. Generally, cell surface expression of TLRs is rather low, varying in monocytes from a few hundred to a few thousand molecules per cell (**Visintin** *et al.*, 2001). TLRs can be either ubiquitous (TLR1), restricted (TLR2, TLR4, and TLR5), or specific (TLR3) as per their cellular expression pattern. TLR1 shows the most ubiquitous expression pattern, showing its possible role as regulator of TLR-mediated signaling (**Spitzer** *et al.*, 2002). TLR3 shows the most restricted expression pattern, and is predominantly present in immature dendritic cells (Muzio *et al.*, 200). Expression of TLRs declines with age, which leads to increased susceptibility of elderly people to infections (**Renshaw *et al.*, 2002**). TLR expression appears to be much higher in farmer's children than in non-farmer's children (**Lauener *et al.*, 2002**), which might again correlate with individual differences in pathogen susceptibility (**Arbour *et al.*, 2000**). TLRs also exhibit specific subcellular expression patterns, reflecting their ability to recognize different microbial ligands, which gain access to the cell at different subcellular sites (**Ahmad *et al.*, 2002).** Phagosome expression of TLR2 and probably also other TLRs presumably enables them to sample the contents of vacuoles for different pathogen-associated molecular patterns, which are internalized by other pattern recognition receptors, like the mannose receptor (**Underhill *et al.*, 1999**). Gewirtz et al. showed that localized expression of TLR5 is responsible for flagellin recognition in epithelial cells of the gastrointestinal tract contributes to the differential response to commensal and pathogenic bacteria (**Gewirtz *et al.*, 2001**).

Future Prospects in TLR Research

TLRs have been implicated as a family of proteins which are involved in induction of innate immune response against microbial insult from surrounding, such as bacteria and virus. Today, a research between innate immunity and cancer is drawing a lot of attention from investigators, and this study actually provides critical information for development of therapeutic strategies against cancer. Recent studies and patents showed TLR expression profile could be one of guidelines for diagnosis of specific cancer. Using TLR agonist or antagonist in combination with antigen isolated from tumor, we can anticipate increasing effect of vaccination and evoking specific innate immunity against cancer. Although TLR can mediate host innate immune system, over-expression of TLRs has been paradoxically found in many tumor cases. Furthermore, it has been demonstrated that TLR-mediated signaling promotes tumor growth, and escape of tumor cells from host immune system has been observed in some cancer models. These studies and observation strongly suggest that biological outcomes induced by high levels of the protein are determined by both inter- and intra-cellular environment. Although recent issues have continuously claimed that specific TLR or signaling molecules in TLR pathway are involved in pathogenesis of cancers, choices of use of either agonist or antagonist for TLR in the context of therapy could not be decided immediately. The study of TLRs is still in early stage, so we need to explore more detailed function of each TLR in different types of cancer. Without that information, one would not be able to develop therapeutic strategies using TLR pathway.

Conclusion

Toll-like receptors comprise a family of pattern recognition receptors. The effects of their activation reach beyond innate immune reactions. Activating dendritic cells and modulating specific immune reactions at the levels of T and B cells link mechanisms of innate and adaptive immunity to elicit an efficient response against the invading pathogen or maintenance of homeostasis. However, TLR involvement in the pathogenesis of neoplastic diseases has also been observed. Some issues concerning the exploitation of TLRs in the treatment of neoplastic diseases still need to be addressed. It is crucial to adequately assess the expression of TLRs on transformed cells and study the biology of TLR signaling, as there are still some discrepancies among researchers about the functionality of TLRs in malignant cells. The functionality of TLRs in transformed cells goes far beyond simple NFêB activation, but should be studied in the context of the tumor environment with its suppressive nature and weak immunogenicity.

References

1. Singh VK, Ducey EJ, Fatanmi OO, Singh PK, Brown DS (2012). CBLB613: a TLR 2/6 agonist, natural lipopeptide of Mycoplasma arginini, as a novel radiation counter measure. *Radiat Res* **177(5):** 628-642.
2. Andersen JM, Al-Khairy D, Ingalls RR (2006). Innate immunity at the mucosal surface: role of toll-like receptor 3 and toll-like receptor 9 in cervical epithelial cell responses to microbial pathogens. *Biol Reprod* **74(5):** 824-831.
3. Pradhan VD, Das S, Surve P, Ghosh K (2012). Toll-like receptors in autoimmunity with special reference to systemic lupus erythematosus. *Indian J Hum Genet* **18(2):** 155-160.
4. Tipping PG (2006). Toll-like receptors: the interface between innate and adaptive immunity. *J Am Soc Nephrol* **17(7):** 1769-1771.
5. Singh VK, Pollard HB (2015). Patents for Toll-like receptor ligands as radiation counter measures for acute radiation syndrome. *Expert Opin Ther Pat* **25(10):** 1085-1092.
6. Kawai T, Akira S (2006). TLR signaling. *Cell Death Differ* **13(5):** 816- 825.
7. Hoebe K, Janssen E, Beutler B (2004). The interface between innate and adaptive immunity. *Nat Immunol* **5(10):** 971-974.
8. Husebye H, Halaas O, Stenmark H, Tunheim G, Sandanger O, et al. (2006). Endocytic pathways regulate Toll-like receptor 4 signaling and link innate and adaptive immunity. *EMBO J* **25(4):** 683-692.
9. Kabelitz D (2007) Expression and function of Toll-like receptors in T lymphocytes. *Curr Opin Immunol* **19(1):** 39-45.
10. Kanzler H, Barrat FJ, Hessel EM, Coffman RL (2007). Therapeutic targeting of innate immunity with Toll-like receptor agonists and antagonists. *Nat Med* **13(5):** 552-559.

11. Yoon SI, Kurnasov O, Natarajan V, Hong M, Gudkov AV (2012). Structural basis of TLR5-flagellin recognition and signaling. *Science* **335(6070):** 859-864.

12. Alderton GK (2012). Signalling: New roles for TLR2. *Nat Rev Immunol* **12(12):** 810-811.

13. Bell JK, Mullen GE, Leifer CA, Mazzoni A, Davies DR, Segal DM (2003). Leucine-rich repeats and pathogen recognition in Toll-like receptors. *Trends Immunol*. **24**: 528-533.

14. Rock FL, Hardiman G, Timans JC, Kastelein RA, Bazan JF (1998). A family of human receptors structurally related to Drosophila Toll. *Proc. Natl. Acad. Sci. USA* **95**: 588–593.

15. Akira S and Takeda K (2005). Toll like receptors in innate immunity. *Intl. Immunol.* **17(1):** 1-14.

16. Banchereau J and Steinman RM (1998). Dendritic cells and the control of immunity. *Nature*, **392:** 245–252.

17. Hosseini AM., Majidi J, Baradaran B, Yousefi M (2015). Toll like receptors in the pathogenesis of autoimmune diseases. *Adv.Pharm Bull.* **5(1):** 605-614.

18. Dadi S, Chhangawala S, Whitlock BM, Franklin RA, Luo CT (2016). Cancer Immunosurveillance by Tissue-Resident Innate Lymphoid Cells and Innate-like T Cells. *Cell* **164(3):** 365-377.

19. Dietsch GN, Randall TD, Gottardo R, Northfelt DW, Ramanathan RK (2015). Late-Stage Cancer Patients Remain Highly Responsive to Immune Activation by the Selective TLR8 Agonist Motolimod (VTX- 2337). *Clin Cancer Res* **21(24):** 5445-5452.

20. Gajewski TF, Schreiber H, Fu YX (2013). Innate and adaptive immune cells in the tumor microenvironment. *Nat Immunol* **14(10):** 1014-1022.

21. Zhang Y, Luo F, Cai Y, Liu N, Wang L (2011). TLR1/TLR2 agonist induces tumor regression by reciprocal modulation of effector and regulatory T cells. *J Immunol* **186(4):** 1963-1969.

22. Vacchelli E, Vitale I, Tartour E, Eggermont A, Sautès-Fridman C (2013). Trial Watch: Anticancer radioimmunotherapy. *Oncoimmunology* **2(9):** e25595.

23. Northfelt DW, Ramanathan RK, Cohen PA, Von Hoff DD, Weiss GJ (2014). A phase I dose-finding study of the novel Toll-like receptor 8 agonist VTX-2337 in adult subjects with advanced solid tumors or lymphoma. *Clin Cancer Res* **20(14):** 3683-3691.

24. Vacchelli E, Eggermont A, Sautès-Fridman C, Galon J, Zitvogel L (2013). Trial Watch: Toll-like receptor agonists for cancer therapy. *Oncoimmunology* **2(8):** e25238.

25. Gearing AJ (2007) Targeting toll-like receptors for drug development: a summary of commercial approaches. *Immunol Cell Biol* **85(6):** 490-494.

26. Visintin A, Mazzoni A, Spitzer JH, Wyllie DH, Dower SK, Segal DM (2001). Regulation of Toll-like receptors in human monocytes and dendritic cells. *J. Immunol* **166:** 249-255.

27. Spitzer JH, Visintin A, Mazzoni A, Kennedy MN, Segal DM (2002). Toll-like receptor 1 inhibits Toll-like receptor 4 signaling in endothelial cells. Eur. *J. Immunol* **32:** 1182-1187.

28. Muzio M, Bosisio D, Polentarutti N, D'Amico G, Stoppacciaro A, Mancinelli R, van't Veer C, Penton-Rol G, Ruco LP, Allavena P, Mantovani A. (2000). Differential expression and regulation of Toll-like receptors (TLR) in human leukocytes: selective expression of TLR3 in dendritic cells. *J. Immunol.* **164:** 5998-6004.

29. Renshaw M, Rockwell J, Engleman C, Gewirtz A, Katz J, Sambhara S (2002). Cutting edge: impaired Toll-like receptor expression and function in aging. *J. Immunol.* **169:** 4697-4701.

30. Lauener RP, Birchler T, Adamski J, Braun-Fahrlander C, Bufe A, Herz U, von Mutius E, Nowak D, Riedler J, Waser M, Sennhauser FH (2002). Expression of CD14 and Toll-like receptor 2 in farmers' and non-farmers' children. *Lancet* **360:** 465-466.

31. Arbour NC, Lorenz E, Schutte BC, Zabner J, Kline JN, Jones M, Frees K, Watt JL, Schwartz DA (2000). TLR4 mutations are associated with endotoxin hyporesponsiveness in humans. *Nat. Genet.* **25:** 187-191.

32. Ahmad-Nejad P, Hacker H, Rutz M, Bauer S, Vabulas RM, Wagner H (2002). Bacterial CpG-DNA and lipopolysaccharides activate Toll-like receptors at distinct cellular compartments. Eur. *J. Immunol.* **32:** 1958-1968.

33. Underhill, DM, Ozinsky A, Hajjar AM, Stevens A, Wilson CB, Bassetti M, Aderem A (1999). The Toll-like receptor 2 is recruited to macrophage phagosomes and discriminates between pathogens. *Nature* **401:** 811-815.

34. Gewirtz, AT, Navas TA, Lyons S, Godowski PJ, Madara JL (2001). Cutting edge: bacterial flagellin activates basolaterally expressed TLR5 to induce epithelial proinflammatory gene expression. *J. Immunol* **167:** 1882-1885.

❑❑❑

3

Enhancing Heterologous Protection Against Porcine Reproductive and Respiratory Syndrome Virus: Challenges and Opportunities

Nadeem Shabir*, Amina Khatun, Salik Nazki, Riaz A Shah, Nazir A Ganai, Syed Shanaz, Mahak Khan, Abrar A Malik, Towseef Akram, Won-Il Kim and Vikas Mahajan

* Division of Animal Biotechnology, Faculty of Veterinary Sciences and Animal Husbandry, Sher-e-Kashmir University of Agricultural Sciences and Technology of Kashmir (SKUAST-K), Srinagar, India E-mail: nadeem.shabir@skuastkashmir.ac.in

Porcine Reproductive & Respiratory Syndrome Virus (PRRSV) belongs to Arteriviridae family, which also includes equine arteritis virus (EAV), lactate dehydrogenase elevating virus (LDV) of mice, and simian haemorrhagic fever virus (SHFV). The genome of PRRSV is single-stranded, positive-sense RNA of nearly 15 kb that encodes 10 open reading frames (ORF): ORF1a, ORF1b, ORF2a, ORF2b and ORFs 3–7, which includes ORF5 and ORF5a (39, 52). ORF1a and ORF1b encode two polyproteins, pp1a and pp1a/b, and the latter is expressed due to ribosomal frame-shifting (28). ORF1 (a and b) code for two large polyproteins that are cleaved into 14 non-structural proteins (37). Pp1a and pp1a/b are proteolytically cleaved into 14 non-structural proteins (Nsp's) by the papain-like cysteine protease (PCP) in Nsp1, poliovirus 3C-like cysteine protease (CP) in Nsp2, and serine protease (SP) in Nsp4. Nsp12 is cleaved through Nsp3 by SP, and Nsp1• and Nsp1ß are generated by PCP, while as Nsp2 is generated by CP (37). Three N-glycosylated minor envelope proteins viz., GP2a, GP3 and GP4 are encoded by ORFs 2a, 3 and 4 encode, respectively, which form heterodimers through disulphide bonds (153). A non-glycosylated minor protein is encoded by ORF2b that lies within ORF2a, (155). ORF-5 and ORF-6 encode two major envelope proteins

GP5 and GP6, respectively which form a heterodimer (77). The GP5-6 heterodimer is believed to play a crucial role in virus assembly through recruitment of other envelope protein heterodimers (153). Moreover, GP5a, encoded by an alternate ORF5, has been recently identified (52). The N protein is expressed from ORF7 and has been reported to contain nuclear localization signals (NLSs) and nuclear export signals (NESs) (117).

PRRSV has been classified into two divergent genotypes viz. European also known as Type 1 and North American, also known as Type 2, that are further sub-divided into at least nine different genetic lineages (83, 92, 121, 123). While high intra-genotypic heterogeneity between strains has been reported, PRRSV has also been demonstrated to show genetic variability after pig-to-pig serial passages (14). The higher genetic variability in turn increases antigenic diversity which translates into diversified immunogenicity of different PRRSVs as evinced by previous studies (41, 125). Consequently, this increasing diversity among PRRSVs not only hinders the comprehension of PRRSV-induced immunity but also poses a serious hurdle for selection of immunogenic strains for vaccine development (82). Currently, a foremost disadvantage of existing PRRS modified live vaccines (MLVs) is that they offer inadequate or no cross-protection, even though solid homologous protection has been reported (82, 95, 100, 120). Killed PRRS vaccines have also been previously used, but they offer limited protection against even homologous viruses (60). It is now generally accepted that strain-specific vaccines cannot fully protect against newly emerging PRRSV outbreaks, whereas multi-strain vaccines have shown more severe clinical signs in pigs (84). Moreover, owing to a considerable variation between PRRSV strains in terms of replication efficiency (53), immune response (41) and neutralizing antibody induction (58), multi-strain vaccines for PRRS do not hold much promise. Conventional methods used in RNA virus vaccine development have been successful in the past, but mutagenesis using a reverse genetics approach might prove to be more efficient (129).

Antibody-mediated Immunological Reaction

1. PRRS virus-specific non-neutralizing antibody response

A good anti-PRRSV antibody response can be calculated, from 7–9 days post-infection (dpi). IgG antibody levels appear to peak at 21–35 dpi in piglets but persist at lower levels thereafter (91). However, there is no role of these antibodies in protection against PRRSV infection (63, 159) which has also been validated by in-vitro studies (159). Interestingly, the passive protection tryouts using initial PRRSV-specific antibodies collected as early as 21 dpi has not been shown to offer passive protection counter to a virulent antibody-matched PRRSV, and instead has been apparently observed to enhance the virulence of the infection (71). Thus, the non-neutralizing antibodies could also be elicit an antibody-dependent enhancement (ADE) of viral copying which has been observed in-vitro and in-vivo (44, 160, 161). This trend is labelled as an amplified internalization of the virus inside macrophages as an outcome of opsonization by non-neutralizing antibodies. As per some reports (13, 151, 160) N protein and GP5 could home the epitopes which are incharge for the induction of antibodies involved in the process of ADE. However, some laboratories have reported contrasting results in detection of ADE in PRRSV infection which have been attributed to 'virus strain or swine macrophage differences' (26). Moreover, the ADE reported in the previous in-vivo studies of PRRSV infection (71) could not rule out the likelihood of augmented pathology caused due to pro-inflammatory cytokines in PRRS co-salted out with IgG fractions. Overall, the role of ADE in the pathogenesis of PRRS is doubtful as has been unfavourably discussed in the previous review (93). More recent efforts have shown that anti-nsp antibodies also are found early after infection (22, 101).

2. PRRSV-specific Neutralizing Antibody Response

Serum virus neutralizing (SVN) antibodies against PRRSV infection usually appear around 21 to 28 dpi or even later (30, 69, 80, 133). However, their onset can be influenced by the strain which is used for the infection, minor alterations of the viral neutralization test or both (30, 58, 133). Cross-neutralization between various of strains PRRSV is thought to be dependent on the homologies of structural proteins (ORFs 2-6) (25, 31, 50, 51, 56, 57, 88, 107, 112, 145). In any instance, NA titres against PRRSV are often low (below 1:32-1:64) in wild-type viruses inoculated pigs (30, 69, 80).

In virus neutralization, major role of ORFs 5-6 has been elucidated in previous studies (43, 50, 51, 95, 108, 111, 115, 150). Also, titers have been reported to demonstrate variability among pigs with a specific strain inoculation (110). Attenuated vaccines induce much lower or in-significant titers of SVN antibodies while inactivated vaccines are most often unable to induce SVN antibodies prior to a challenge (29, 57, 166). However, it has been reported that the inactivated vaccines upon challenge might harvest NA responses if they go through a previously optimized inactivation process (UV irradiation or treatment with binary ethylenimine) which, however, does not distort the structure of NE, and if they are used with an appropriate adjuvant (144).

Multiple viral targets for SVN antibodies have been described in previous reports, including GP3(57), GP4 (20, 43, 88, 150), GP5 (13, 57, 108, 150) and M proteins (13, 59). However, but it is generally believed that the virus's core neutralization epitope (NE) is possibly harboured by GP5 (102, 109). It has also been reported that PRRSV infection can be blocked by SVN antibodies by inhibiting the collaboration of the virus with the internalization receptor sialoadhesin (Sn) on macrophages (26, 139, 143). Lately, the interaction of GP4 and GP2a with CD163 has been demonstrated (21). The deferred development of SVN antibodies and their low titers in immunized pigs has been the focus of many studies, lately. One of such studies has suggested that variable expression of antigen presentation molecules or poor cytokine stimulation could cause deferred recruitment of cells from the acquired part of immune system that could lead to delayed SVN antibody response to PRRSV (15, 40). One of the other hypotheses attributes the delayed SVN antibody response to the presence of a decoy epitope in PRRSV (102). In this line of thought an immunodominant epitope would be located close to the NE of GP5 and would thus, divert the immune system. An introduction of pan-DR helper T-cell epitope between NE of GP5 and the predicted decoy epitope increased SVN antibody response was observed in a mouse model which indicates the significance of the decoy epitope (36). Amount of glycosylation in or around NE is one of the other vital conditions. Around 3 glycosylation sites might be observed in genotype I strains in or adjoining the GP5 NE, while as 4 probable glycosylation sites for genotype II strains might be found. Glycosylation patterns have been found to vary among different genotype II PRRSV isolates as observed in previous studies (34). It has been observed that the loss of two upstream glycosylations in an isolate (HV-1) resulted in higher levels of SVN antibodies than the glycosylated strains (*i.e.,* VR-2332) which were subsequently confirmed by the generation of mutants lacking some glycosylation in other studies (5). Thus, the glycosylations loss in GP5 ectodomain could increase the homologous and cross-protective immunity of PRRSV vaccines.

Role of Innate, Adaptive & Regulatory Immunity in Protection

1. Innate immune response to PRRSV infection

Production of type I interferons (IFNs), IFN-α and IFN-β, by virus-infected cells is the most efficient innate anti-viral immune response which by the expression of several interferon-roused genes induces an antiviral state (7). In PRRSV infection, type I IFNs (α and β) have been showed to restrict PRRSV replication in vitro (70, 103, 118), which suggests their significant anti-PRRSV function. However, previous studies also indicate that PRRSV either induces insignificant amounts of interferon IFN-α or inhibits the cytokine (3, 11, 46), while as other studies have demonstrated virus strain-dependent induction/ inhibition of IFN-α in enriched plasmacytoid dendritic cells (pDCs) and strain specific IFN-α-induction and sensitivity to the cytokine in swine PAMs (8, 65). Swine transmissible gastroenteritis virus (TGEV) and porcine respiratory coronavirus (PRCV) induced high level of IFN-α while as PRRSV appears to inhibit synthesis of type I IFNs in pigs (3, 11). The IFN-inducing ability of PRRSV has been estimated to be at least 159-fold lower than that of PRCV (11). PRRSV infection of pulmonary alveolar macrophages (PAMs) does not lead to IFN-a production (3).

Barring the modulation of the IFN organization, PRRSV also seems to control other cytokines. The pro-inflammatory cytokines *viz.*, TNF-α, IL-1, and IL-8 have been the attention of most studies. PRRSV has been reported to also inhibit TNF-α production in-vitro and in-vivo (42, 70) and its induction by LPS and PMA in porcine PAMs cultures (48, 70), however, a recent study (47) demonstrated differential TNF-α production by a high and low pathogenic PRRSV strain in swine PAMs. Other studies had similar observations in bronchoalveolar lavages (BAL) of PRRSV-infected pigs (135, 142). However, IL-1 responses were identified in not only these two studies, but in many others as well (62, 140). Further, some in-vitro studies with PAM (2, 17), PBMC (1) or in-vivo/ex-vivo studies (1, 17, 89, 140) demonstrated induction of TNF-α mRNA accumulation or detected the cytokine by flow cytometry or ELISA. Numerous studies have shown that PRRSV induces IL-8 (1, 68, 135) while as vitro or ex-vivo IL-6 production has been shown by some studies (68, 106, 140), however, other studies did not observe it (29, 30).

2. T cell immunity in PRRSV Infection

Because of their vital role in development and regulation of antigen-specific immune responses, T cells play a significant role in several facets of anti-PRRSV immunity, including tutoring and activation of B cells, determination of the cytokine locale in the environment of antigen presentation, function of cytotoxic effector to terminate the infected cells, and immune response regulation to govern inflammation and screen the autoimmune reactions (73).

CD3, CD4, and CD8 along with secretion of interferon-gamma (IFN-γ) are primary phenotypic characteristics of swine T cell subpopulations. Previous reports suggest that porcine have a considerable inhabitation of mature CD4/CD8 double-positive T cells that also represent memory T cells (167). It has further been reported that these cells have an capability to produce IFN-ã and restrict to the sites of inflammation, which indicates their important role in mediating protective immunity (166). The cell-mediated immune response in PRRSV infection is nearly analogous to the cytokine response. A temporary decrease of $CD4^+$ T cells has been observed in blood after 3-7days after PRRSV infection, which after 7-14 days post infection (DPI) return to normal (99, 124). Also, higher $CD8^+$ T cells have been reported 4-5 weeks post infection (4, 55, 124). $CD4^+$ T cells have been demonstrated to be the major proliferating effector cell (9) while as IFNã has been used as a marker of T_{H1} polarization of helper T cell responses in PRRSV infection (81, 156). The cytotoxic T cell activity against PRRSV-infected macrophages develops very slowly and was not identified until 49 DPI (19). In another report, a low virus-specific $CD8^+$ T cells secreting IFNγ has been found that was confirmed with a minimal CTL response, however, in the same study it was observed that immune triggering was influenced by isolate and not route of administration (38).

3. Regulation of Immune Response in PRRSV Infection

Many studies in the past have suggested interleukin-10 (IL-10) up-regulation in PRRSV infection as one of the major immune-evasive strategies adopted by the virus (16, 29, 69, 105, 128, 149), however, other study demonstrated variable levels of IL-10 induced by different PRRSV strains (29). Among these strategies, induction of IL-10 and regulatory T cells (Tregs) are believed to play an important role in determining the immunological and clinical outcomes of PRRS infection (72, 80, 82, 132). Generally, $CD4^+/CD25^+/FoxP3^+$ is the accepted phenotype of IL-10 producing regulatory T cells (Treg) or TGF-β and that are able to downregulate or prevent proliferation or effector abilities of other T-cells upon stimulation with a recall antigen. These characteristics have also been shown to apply to porcine Treg (54).

PRRSV infection reportedly causes increase in the frequency of TGF-β producing putative regulatory T cells (Tregs) (127). In infected dendritic cells, Type 1 PRRSV strains induce IL-10 production, but co-culture with lymphocytes does not induce Treg cells or TGF-β production (125). By contrast, dendritic cells infected with Type 2 PRRSV can increase Tregs and stimulate TGF-β production (126). Recent work indicates that monocyte-derived dendritic cells infected with either of the types of PRRSV *viz.,* Type 1 or Type 2 do not elevate the frequency or proliferation of $CD4^+$ $Foxp3^+$ regulatory T cells in an in-vitro co-culture system (114). PRRSV induction of Tregs with suppressive activity occurs both in-vitro and in-vivo (154).

Role of Structural Genes in PRRSV-elicited Immune Response

1. Location and roles of neutralizing epitopes in protection

GP5 and M form the major envelope proteins of PRRSV (85, 97) and the two envelope proteins form a heterodimeric complex with each other that is linked by a disulfide bond (77). Much as was demonstrated for LDV and EAV, both GP5 and M are thought to cross the viral envelope three times and have only a small extravirion domain and a longer intravirion domain (23, 35). It has been reported that GP5 is the most variable structural protein, and the predicted ectodomain following signal sequence cleavage is around 32 residues (134). Two hypervariable regions surround a quite conserved region within these 32 amino acids, which contains the completely conserved cysteine disulfide-linked to M and two potential N-glycosylation sites (75, 111). While the N-terminal sequence has been called as a decoy epitope (non-neutralizing), the conserved domain has been demonstrated to host a neutralization domain (71, 72, 79, 102, 109, 111, 131). However, being surrounded by complex oligosaccharides the conserved domain is masked from neutralizing antibodies (102, 110). Also, the M protein, which is assumed to assemble all virion components together, has been demonstrated to have a role in neutralization (13, 27).

A significant analysis on major targets *viz.*, GP4 and GP5 of SVN antibodies, with an importance positioned on GP5, was initiated after earlier reports indicated that GP5 and GP4 specific monoclonal antibodies (141) possessed PRRSV-neutralizing capacity. Majortiy of previous reports suggested that GP5 hosts the major neutralizing epitope(s) (107, 108, 150, 157), besides which an additional neutralizing epitope was documented by a monoclonal anti-body on the envelope's GP4 (141, 157), and one more on the envelope protein M (157). Lately, it has also been demonstrated that the broadly neutralizing activity mediated by polyclonal swine antibody could be influenced by a solo amino acid within the M protein (137). Some reports have previously established that the chief neutralizing epitope was positioned on the GP5 ectodomain which encompasses amino acids 37 to 44 as the fundamental of the chief neutralizing epitope (102, 111). Additionally, neutralizing epitopes have also been shown to be harboured by two of the minor glycoproteins (GP3 and GP4) (20, 57, 85, 130, 145, 148, 164). These minor glycoprotein might play a role in neutralization of some or all PRRSV strains; however, there is not much information regarding the functions of these proteins. (32, 113, 152).

2. Viral epitopes of T cell immunity

Immune assays that are usually used to assess antigen-specific responses have been used to investigate cell-mediated immunity targets of PRRSV antigens. Induction of proliferative responses have been observed by incubation of PBMC from pigs infected with PRRSV in the presence of envelope glycoproteins *viz.*, (GP) 2 and 5, and matrix (M) protein (10). Using an IFN-γ secreting-cell ELISPOT assay immunodominant epitopes, including conserved amino acid regions at residues 117–131 and 149–163 were evaluated i8n GP5 (12, 146). Further, in N and GP5 of Type 1 PRRS V, conserved T cell epitopes were identified, with the GP5 epitope analogous to epitopes reported in Type 2 PRRSV (31). Also, in a Chinese highly pathogenic PRRSV strain, using IFN-ã ELISPOT four conserved T cell peptides have been classified in its matrix (membrane) protein (149). Conserved epitopes in Type 2 PRRSV were recognized in nsp2, nsp9 and nsp10 in the non-structural protein repertoire that enhanced the antigen-specific proliferation and secretion of IFN-γ (12, 104). Peptides, few of which repressed IFN-γ responses, but stimulating secretion of IL-10 were also observed in PBMC stimulated with mitogen. Pigs homozygous for

SLA haplotypes have been observed to be low IFN-γ responders, although the implication of this study was not pursued (12). A recent study has demonstrated the use of PRRSV M and NSP5 peptides in hydrophobic chitosin-based particulate formulations as vaccine candidate T-cell antigens (90).

Approaches to Improve Protective Immunity

1. Chimeric PRRSVs

Until now, using reverse genetics technology, over 14 infectious clones of type I and type II PRRSV have been developed, and this approach can be further employed to construct safe and efficacious chimeric vaccines against PRRSV (45, 158). A recent study has revealed that vaccine chimeras between MN-184 and licensed MLV (Ingelvac® PRRS MLV) could attenuate clinical signs in pigs challenged with virulent viruses (33). The infectious cDNA clones have been used by a number of researchers to generate viable chimeric arterivirus by replacing genes of one PRRS strain for those of another strain or other non-PRRS arterivirus. The VR-2332 infectious clone as a backbone has been used to study the role of individual envelope proteins of GP2 through M for cross-neutralization (59). Susceptibility to serum neutralization and rapid induction of robust neutralizing antibodies in pigs is determined to be high in case of PRRSV-01 strain. The two N-linked glycosylation sites each in GP3 and GP5 have been found to be absent in structural genes of PRRSV-01. The missing glycans for neutralization were replaced to determine the significance of GP3 and GP5 genes from PRRSV-01 (147). The genetic compatibility and viral-specific phenotypes like neutralization, virulence, and pathogenesis have been studied using intra-genotypic or inter-genotypic gene-swapping methods between EAV and PRRSV. Nine chimeric EAVs containing individual ORF5 from different isolates have been constructed to check the neutralization response (6). The viral gene swapping technique of genes from a non-virulent, mitigated strain of PRRSV into a virulent infectious cDNA clone (FL-12) have been used to help assign contributions of these genes to virulence in the pig. Virulence seemed to be critically decreased, when the chimeric viruses containing ORF 5 or nsps 3–8 from the vaccine virus were used. While as virulence was not much affected when ORF 2 and nsps 1–3 and 10–12 were used as compared to virus formed by the FL-12 parental cDNA clone (61). The dominant Korean field strain LMY was recently used to generate a chimeric infectious clone by replacing the structural genes of the FL-12 clone (64). On swapping the envelope proteins representing GP2 through GP5 of genotype I in that of genotype II backbone proved to be fully practical (136). A major hurdle for producing a broadly-protective vaccine against genetically diverse field strains is the widespread antigenic and genetic heterogeneity of PRRSV (49, 82). At least 9 distinct genetic lineages within Type 2 PRRSV and 3 subtypes within Type 1 PRRSV have been observed (94, 122). A new virus containing a new GP3 gene, produced by randomly shuffling GP3 sequences of immunologically diverse strains of PRRSV and incorporating it in the infectious clone have been used to enhance the cross neutralization (165). A broad spectrum of cross-neutralizing antibodies has been observed in the rescued virus after the breeding of GP4 and M gene (164). The phenomenon of appearance of certain codon pairs in a higher frequency as compared to other synonymous codon pairs for the identical amino acid is referred to as codon-pair bias (18). Synthetic attenuated virus engineering (SAVE), through codon pairs deoptimization of the major envelope gene, was used to efficiently attenuate PRRSV. The major gain is the rapid nature of the method to develop vaccines against newly emerged PRRSV strains as compared to the time consuming traditional virus attenuation methods. Moreover, SAVE approach helps to retain the antigenicity of the attenuated vaccine virus as that of the wild type and thus can be effectively used to design vaccines against diverse strains of PRRSV.

2. PRRSVs engineered to express cytokines

Previous research has suggested that PRRSV modulates innate or regulatory immune response which leads to delayed activation of the adaptive immune system eventually aiding the virus replication in pigs. Recently, there have been some efforts to express certain cytokines from a new subgenomic (sg) RNA engineered between the ORF1ab and ORF2a/b. One of such engineered viruses was generated from P129-based vector that was engineered to express various porcine interferons (IFNs α1, β, δ3 and ω) that, however, displayed reduced growth which was similar to the effect of adding the exogenous interferon protein (119). Similarly, P129-based vector was engineered to express IL-1β which was reported to show attenuated virulence in pigs and upregulation of some cytokines like IL-1β, Il-4 and IFN-γ. Also, an HuN4-F112-based vector was used to express porcine granulocyte-macrophage colony stimulating factor (GM-CSF) using transcriptional regulatory sequence (TRS) 6 and the virus generated was found to be stable, expressed GM-CSF as potential vaccine adjuvant and induced a significant higher cellular immune response and reduced the persistent infection (66). Recently, IL-4 was cloned and engineered in CH-1R strain of PRRSV to express IL-4 using transcriptional regulatory sequence (TRS) 6, and the pigs infected with this virus were observed to have higher IL-4 levels in blood and higher $CD4^+$, $CD8^+$ double positive cells (67).

3. Unwinding Overlaps Between Open Reading Frames (ORFs)

The successful development of infectious clones of PRRSV (36, 86, 98, 99, 138, 163) have opened new possibilities for molecular dissection of the arteriviral RNA replication and transcription. Development of genetically engineered vaccines against PRRSV could be one of the ways to tackle the PRRSV as the infectious clones provide us with powerful tools to manipulate PRRSV genome through reverse genetic system (RGS) that provides an excellent platform for functional dissection of arteriviral structural proteins (162). One of the major hurdles, however, faced is the variable lengths of overlapping coding sequences shared by adjacent. As an example, ORF3/4 share a 255 nt long overlapping region in Type I PRRSV, while 15 and 10 nt span the coding regions between ORF5/6 and ORF6/7, respectively (83, 87, 96). Previous studies have shown that while the specific collection of the overlapping regions for EAV structural proteins was also indispensable for viral infection, unwinding the overlaps between ORF4/5, ORF5/6, and ORF4/5/6 in EAV infectious clones was possible to rescue virus from transfected cells when overlapping regions between (24). Previous studies on PRRSV has successfully attempted to unwind the overlaps between ORFs 5/6 and 6/7 (162); however, there have not been any studies that have demonstrated the successful removal of ORF2/3 or ORF3/4 overlaps.

4. Enhancement of T cell-mediated immune response

Previous reports have suggested that a sustained effect on the intensity of cell the cell-mediated immune response was observed after the delivery of IFN-α cDNA (81). Similarly, a transient increase in the frequency of PRRSV-specific IFN-γ secreting cells (SCs) was observed after the introduction of the type I interferon analogues like poly I: C, a synthetic double stranded RNA. However, it has to be noted that poly I: C has not been found as effective as the IFN-α encoding plasmid delivered with vaccine for the augmentation of IFN-γ response to

PRRSV. The previous studies have established that significance of IL-12 or IFN-α during PRRSV infection after the introduction of either IL-12 or IFN-α during vaccination augmented the intensity of the IFN-γ response to PRRSV in directing the *in-vivo* differentiation of swine Th1 cells (80, 156).

Enhancement of early IFN-γ cellular immunity through co-administration of adjuvant with modified-live PRRSV has also been observed (76). The ability of IFN-γ it inhibit the PRRSV replication in MARC-145 (116) and porcine alveolar macrophages (PAMs) suggests (9) could suggest its possible role in mediating protective immune response against PRRSV infection. Previous reports have indicated an association between frequency of IFN-γ SCs and protective immunity against PRRSV (16, 74, 78). Improved T cell mediated IFN-γ response after vaccination is one of the major factors in evaluating the advancement of protective efficacy of PRRS vaccines. Nevertheless, the best way to assess the protective immunity induced by the PRRSV vaccine would be the health condition of animals, immunity and its ability to lessen the PRRSV replication in an infection challenge model.

Conclusion

Due to its highly mutating nature, PRRSV has been continuously evolving and has diversified into number of lineages and sub-lineages. This diversity of the virus becomes one of the major hurdles in PRRS vaccinology, since the currently used modified live vaccines (MLVs) against PRRSV only offer homologous protection and lack or offer limited cross-protection. Another major hurdle to PRRSV vaccinology is the modulation of innate immune response by PRRSV which results in delayed activation of its adaptive arm leading to persistence of the virus in hosts for longer periods. Most of the current studies focus on enhancing the protective immune responses by construction of chimera among diverse strains of PRRSVs. The major goal is to attain heterogeneity of neutralizing epitopes in the vaccine candidate to offer broad cross-protection. However, it seems that the protective immunity in PRRSV infection can be improved by enhancement of the T-cell mediated immune response also which has lead the researchers to develop PRRSV infectious clones expressing certain cytokines like type-I IFNs, IL-4, IL-1β, etc. and adjuvant like GM-CSF. Therefore, the future PRRSV vaccines should entail heterogeneous neutralizing epitopes as well as appropriate adjuvant to enhance the protection.

References

1. Aasted, B., P. Bach, J. Nielsen, and P. Lind. 2002. Cytokine profiles in peripheral blood mononuclear cells and lymph node cells from piglets infected in utero with porcine reproductive and respiratory syndrome virus. Clin Diagn Lab Immunol **9:** 1229-1234.
2. Ait-Ali, T., A. D. Wilson, D. G. Westcott, M. Clapperton, M. Waterfall, M. A. Mellencamp, T. W. Drew, S. C. Bishop, and A. L. Archibald. 2007. Innate immune responses to replication of porcine reproductive and respiratory syndrome virus in isolated Swine alveolar macrophages. Viral Immunol **20:** 105-118.
3. Albina, E., C. Carrat, and B. Charley. 1998. Interferon-alpha response to swine arterivirus (PoAV), the porcine reproductive and respiratory syndrome virus. J Interferon Cytokine Res **18:**485-490.
4. Albina, E., L. Piriou, E. Hutet, R. Cariolet, and R. L'Hospitalier. 1998. Immune responses in pigs infected with porcine reproductive and respiratory syndrome virus (PRRSV). Vet Immunol Immunopathol **61:** 49-66.
5. Ansari, I. H., B. Kwon, F. A. Osorio, and A. K. Pattnaik. 2006. Influence of N-linked glycosylation of porcine reproductive and respiratory syndrome virus GP5 on virus infectivity, antigenicity, and ability to induce neutralizing antibodies. J Virol **80:** 3994-4004.
6. Balasuriya, U. B., J. C. Dobbe, H. W. Heidner, V. L. Smalley, A. Navarrette, E. J. Snijder, and N.J. MacLachlan. 2004. Characterization of the neutralization determinants of equine arteritis virus using recombinant chimeric viruses and site-specific mutagenesis of an infectious cDNA clone. Virology **321:** 235-246.
7. Baum, A., and A. Garcia-Sastre. 2010. Induction of type I interferon by RNA viruses: cellular receptors and their substrates. Amino Acids **38:** 1283-1299.
8. Baumann, A., E. Mateu, M. P. Murtaugh, and A. Summerfield. 2013. Impact of genotype 1 and 2 of porcine reproductive and respiratory syndrome viruses on interferon-alpha responses by plasmacytoid dendritic cells. Vet Res **44:** 33.
9. Bautista, E. M., and T. W. Molitor. 1997. Cell-mediated immunity to porcine reproductive and respiratory syndrome virus in swine. Viral Immunol **10:** 83-94.
10. Bautista, E. M., and T. W. Molitor. 1999. IFN gamma inhibits porcine reproductive and respiratory syndrome virus replication in macrophages. Arch Virol **144:** 1191-1200.

11. Buddaert, W., K. Van Reeth, and M. Pensaert. 1998. In-vivo and in-vitro interferon (IFN) studies with the porcine reproductive and respiratory syndrome virus (PRRSV). Adv Exp Med Biol **440:** 461-467.

12. Burgara-Estrella, A., I. Diaz, I. M. Rodriguez-Gomez, S. E. Essler, J. Hernandez, and E. Mateu. 2013. Predicted peptides from non-structural proteins of porcine reproductive and respiratory syndrome virus are able to induce IFN-gamma and IL-10. Viruses **5:** 663-677.

13. Cancel-Tirado, S. M., R. B. Evans, and K. J. Yoon. 2004. Monoclonal antibody analysis of porcine reproductive and respiratory syndrome virus epitopes associated with antibody-dependent enhancement and neutralization of virus infection. Vet Immunol Immunopathol **102:** 249-262.

14. Chang, C. C., K. J. Yoon, J. J. Zimmerman, K. M. Harmon, P. M. Dixon, C. M. Dvorak, and M. P. Murtaugh. 2002. Evolution of porcine reproductive and respiratory syndrome virus during sequential passages in pigs. J Virol **76:** 4750-4763.

15. Chang, H. C., Y. T. Peng, H. L. Chang, H. C. Chaung, and W. B. Chung. 2008. Phenotypic and functional modulation of bone marrow-derived dendritic cells by porcine reproductive and respiratory syndrome virus. Vet Microbiol **129:** 281-293.

16. Charerntantanakul, W., R. Platt, and J. A. Roth. 2006. Effects of porcine reproductive and respiratory syndrome virus-infected antigen-presenting cells on T cell activation and antiviral cytokine production. Viral Immunol **19:** 646-661.

17. Choi, C., W. S. Cho, B. Kim, and C. Chae. 2002. Expression of Interferon-gamma and tumour necrosis factor-alpha in pigs experimentally infected with Porcine Reproductive and Respiratory Syndrome Virus (PRRSV). J Comp Pathol **127:** 106-113.

18. Coleman, J. R., D. Papamichail, S. Skiena, B. Futcher, E. Wimmer, and S. Mueller. 2008. Virus attenuation by genome-scale changes in codon pair bias. Science **320:** 1784-1787.

19. Costers, S., D. J. Lefebvre, B. Goddeeris, P. L. Delputte, and H. J. Nauwynck. 2009. Functional impairment of PRRSV-specific peripheral CD3+CD8high cells. Vet Res **40:** 46.

20. Costers, S., D. J. Lefebvre, J. Van Doorsselaere, M. Vanhee, P. L. Delputte, and H. J. Nauwynck. 2010. GP4 of porcine reproductive and respiratory syndrome virus contains a neutralizing epitope that is susceptible to immunoselection in-vitro. Arch Virol **155:** 371-378.

21. Das, P. B., P. X. Dinh, I. H. Ansari, M. de Lima, F. A. Osorio, and A. K. Pattnaik. 2010. The minor envelope glycoproteins GP2a and GP4 of porcine reproductive and respiratory syndrome virus interact with the receptor CD163. J Virol **84:** 1731-1740.

22. de Lima, M., A. K. Pattnaik, E. F. Flores, and F. A. Osorio. 2006. Serologic marker candidates identified among B-cell linear epitopes of Nsp2 and structural proteins of a North American strain of porcine reproductive and respiratory syndrome virus. Virology **353:** 410-421.

23. de Vries, A. A., E. D. Chirnside, M. C. Horzinek, and P. J. Rottier. 1992. Structural proteins of equine arteritis virus. J Virol **66:** 6294-6303.

24. de Vries, A. A., A. L. Glaser, M. J. Raamsman, C. A. de Haan, S. Sarnataro, G. J. Godeke, and P. J. Rottier. 2000. Genetic manipulation of equine arteritis virus using full-length cDNA clones: separation of overlapping genes and expression of a foreign epitope. Virology **270:** 84-97.

25. Dea, S., C. A. Gagnon, H. Mardassi, B. Pirzadeh, and D. Rogan. 2000. Current knowledge on the structural proteins of porcine reproductive and respiratory syndrome (PRRS) virus: comparison of the North American and European isolates. Arch Virol **145:** 659-688.

26. Delputte, P. L., P. Meerts, S. Costers, and H. J. Nauwynck. 2004. Effect of virus-specific antibodies on attachment, internalization and infection of porcine reproductive and respiratory syndrome virus in primary macrophages. Vet Immunol Immunopathol **102:** 179-188.

27. Delputte, P. L., N. Vanderheijden, H. J. Nauwynck, and M. B. Pensaert. 2002. Involvement of the matrix protein in attachment of porcine reproductive and respiratory syndrome virus to a heparinlike receptor on porcine alveolar macrophages. J Virol **76:** 4312-4320.

28. den Boon, J. A., E. J. Snijder, E. D. Chirnside, A. A. de Vries, M. C. Horzinek, and W. J. Spaan. 1991. Equine arteritis virus is not a togavirus but belongs to the coronaviruslike superfamily. J Virol **65:** 2910-2920.

29. Diaz, I., L. Darwich, G. Pappaterra, J. Pujols, and E. Mateu. 2006. Different European-type vaccines against porcine reproductive and respiratory syndrome virus have different immunological properties and confer different protection to pigs. Virology **351:** 249-259.

30. Diaz, I., L. Darwich, G. Pappaterra, J. Pujols, and E. Mateu. 2005. Immune responses of pigs after experimental infection with a European strain of Porcine reproductive and respiratory syndrome virus. Journal of General Virology **86:** 1943-1951.

31. Diaz, I., J. Pujols, L. Ganges, M. Gimeno, L. Darwich, M. Domingo, and E. Mateu. 2009. In-silico prediction and ex-vivo evaluation of potential T-cell epitopes in glycoproteins 4 and 5 and nucleocapsid protein of genotype-I (European) of porcine reproductive and respiratory syndrome virus. Vaccine **27:** 5603-5611.

32. Du, Y., A. K. Pattnaik, C. Song, D. Yoo, and G. Li. 2012. Glycosyl-phosphatidylinositol (GPI)-anchored membrane association of the porcine reproductive and respiratory syndrome virus GP4 glycoprotein and its co-localization with CD163 in lipid rafts. Virology **424:** 18-32.

33. Ellingson, J. S., Y. Wang, S. Layton, J. Ciacci-Zanella, M. B. Roof, and K. S. Faaberg. 2010. Vaccine efficacy of porcine reproductive and respiratory syndrome virus chimeras. Vaccine **28:** 2679-2686.

34. Faaberg, K. S., J. D. Hocker, M. M. Erdman, D. L. Harris, E. A. Nelson, M. Torremorell, and P. G. Plagemann. 2006. Neutralizing antibody responses of pigs infected with natural GP5 N-glycan mutants of porcine reproductive and respiratory syndrome virus. Viral Immunol **19:** 294-304.

35. Faaberg, K. S., and P. G. Plagemann. 1995. The envelope proteins of lactate dehydrogenase-elevating virus and their membrane topography. Virology **212:** 512-525.

36. Fang, L., Y. Jiang, S. Xiao, C. Niu, H. Zhang, and H. Chen. 2006. Enhanced immunogenicity of the modified GP5 of porcine reproductive & respiratory syndrome virus. Virus Genes **32:** 5-11.

37. Fang, Y., and E. J. Snijder. 2010. The PRRSV replicase: exploring the multifunctionality of an intriguing set of non-structural proteins. Virus Res **154:** 61-76.

38. Ferrari, L., P. Martelli, R. Saleri, E. De Angelis, V. Cavalli, M. Bresaola, M. Benetti, and P. Borghetti. 2013. Lymphocyte activation as cytokine gene expression and secretion is related to the porcine reproductive and respiratory syndrome virus (PRRSV) isolate after in-vitro homologous and heterologous recall of peripheral blood mononuclear cells (PBMC) from pigs vaccinated and exposed to natural infection. Vet Immunol Immunopathol **151:** 193-206.

39. Firth, A. E., J. C. Zevenhoven-Dobbe, N. M. Wills, Y. Y. Go, U. B. Balasuriya, J. F. Atkins, E. J. Snijder, and C. C. Posthuma. 2011.

Discovery of a small arterivirus gene that overlaps the GP5 coding sequence and is important for virus production. Journal of General Virology **92:** 1097-1106.

40. Flores-Mendoza, L., E. Silva-Campa, M. Resendiz, F. A. Osorio, and J. Hernandez. 2008. Porcine reproductive and respiratory syndrome virus infects mature porcine dendritic cells and up-regulates interleukin-10 production. Clinical and Vaccine Immunology **15:** 720-725.

41. Gimeno, M., L. Darwich, I. Diaz, E. de la Torre, J. Pujols, M. Martin, S. Inumaru, E. Cano, M. Domingo, M. Montoya, and E. Mateu. 2011. Cytokine profiles and phenotype regulation of antigen presenting cells by genotype-I porcine reproductive and respiratory syndrome virus isolates. Vet Res **42:** 9.

42. Gomez-Laguna, J., F. J. Salguero, F. J. Pallares, and L. Carrasco. 2013. Immunopathogenesis of porcine reproductive and respiratory syndrome in the respiratory tract of pigs. Vet J **195:** 148-155.

43. Gonin, P., B. Pirzadeh, C. A. Gagnon, and S. Dea. 1999. Seroneutralization of porcine reproductive and respiratory syndrome virus correlates with antibody response to the GP5 major envelope glycoprotein. J Vet Diagn Invest **11:** 20-26.

44. Gu, W., L. Guo, H. Yu, J. Niu, M. Huang, X. Luo, R. Li, Z. Tian, L. Feng, and Y. Wang. 2015. Involvement of CD16 in antibody-dependent enhancement of porcine reproductive and respiratory syndrome virus infection. Journal of General Virology **96:**1712-1722.

45. Han, M., and D. Yoo. 2014. Engineering the PRRS virus genome: Updates and perspectives. Vet Microbiol **174:** 279-295.

46. Han, M., and D. Yoo. 2014. Modulation of innate immune signaling by non-structural protein 1 (nsp1) in the family Arteriviridae. Virus Res **194:** 100-109.

47. He, Q., Y. Li, L. Zhou, X. Ge, X. Guo, and H. Yang. 2015. Both Nsp1beta and Nsp11 are responsible for differential TNF-alpha production induced by porcine reproductive and respiratory syndrome virus strains with different pathogenicity in vitro. Virus Res **201:** 32-40.

48. Hou, J., L. Wang, W. He, H. Zhang, and W. H. Feng. 2012. Highly pathogenic porcine reproductive and respiratory syndrome virus impairs LPS- and poly(I:C)-stimulated tumor necrosis factor-alpha release by inhibiting ERK signaling pathway. Virus Res **167:** 106-111.

49. Huang, Y. W., and X. J. Meng. 2010. Novel strategies and approaches to develop the next generation of vaccines against porcine reproductive and respiratory syndrome virus (PRRSV). Virus Res **154:** 141-149.

50. Jiang, W., P. Jiang, Y. Li, J. Tang, X. Wang, and S. Ma. 2006. Recombinant adenovirus expressing GP5 and M fusion proteins of porcine reproductive and respiratory syndrome virus induce both humoral and cell-mediated immune responses in mice. Vet Immunol Immunopathol **113:** 169-180.

51. Jiang, Y., S. Xiao, L. Fang, X. Yu, Y. Song, C. Niu, and H. Chen. 2006. DNA vaccines co-expressing GP5 and M proteins of porcine reproductive and respiratory syndrome virus (PRRSV) display enhanced immunogenicity. Vaccine **24:** 2869-2879.

52. Johnson, C. R., T. F. Griggs, J. Gnanandarajah, and M. P. Murtaugh. 2011. Novel structural protein in porcine reproductive and respiratory syndrome virus encoded by an alternative ORF5 present in all arteriviruses. Journal of General Virology **92:** 1107-1116.

53. Johnson, W., M. Roof, E. Vaughn, J. Christopher-Hennings, C. R. Johnson, and M. P. Murtaugh. 2004. Pathogenic and humoral immune responses to porcine reproductive and respiratory syndrome virus (PRRSV) are related to viral load in acute infection. Vet Immunol Immunopathol **102:** 233-247.

54. Kaser, T., W. Gerner, S. E. Hammer, M. Patzl, and A. Saalmuller. 2008. Detection of Foxp3 protein expression in porcine T lymphocytes. Vet Immunol Immunopathol **125:** 92-101.

55. Kawashima, K., M. Narita, and S. Yamada. 1999. Changes in macrophage and lymphocyte subpopulations of lymphoid tissues from pigs infected with the porcine reproductive and respiratory syndrome virus (PRRSV). Vet Immunol Immunopathol **71:** 257-262.

56. Kim, W. I., J. J. Kim, S. H. Cha, W. H. Wu, V. Cooper, R. Evans, E. J. Choi, and K. J. Yoon. 2013. Significance of genetic variation of PRRSV ORF5 in virus neutralization and molecular determinants corresponding to cross neutralization among PRRS viruses. Vet Microbiol **162:** 10-22.

57. Kim, W. I., J. J. Kim, S. H. Cha, and K. J. Yoon. 2008. Different biological characteristics of wild-type porcine reproductive and respiratory syndrome viruses and vaccine viruses and identification of the corresponding genetic determinants. J Clin Microbiol **46:** 1758-1768.

58. Kim, W. I., D. S. Lee, W. Johnson, M. Roof, S. H. Cha, and K. J. Yoon. 2007. Effect of genotypic and biotypic differences among PRRS viruses on the serologic assessment of pigs for virus infection. Vet Microbiol **123:** 1-14.

59. Kim, W. I., and K. J. Yoon. 2008. Molecular assessment of the role of envelope-associated structural proteins in cross neutralization among different PRRS viruses. Virus Genes **37:** 380-391.

60. Kimman, T. G., L. A. Cornelissen, R. J. Moormann, J. M. Rebel, and N. Stockhofe-Zurwieden. 2009. Challenges for porcine reproductive and respiratory syndrome virus (PRRSV) vaccinology. Vaccine **27:** 3704-3718.

61. Kwon, B., I. H. Ansari, A. K. Pattnaik, and F. A. Osorio. 2008. Identification of virulence determinants of porcine reproductive and respiratory syndrome virus through construction of chimeric clones. Virology **380:** 371-378.

62. Labarque, G., S. Van Gucht, H. Nauwynck, K. Van Reeth, and M. Pensaert. 2003. Apoptosis in the lungs of pigs infected with porcine reproductive and respiratory syndrome virus and associations with the production of apoptogenic cytokines. Vet Res **34:** 249-260.

63. Labarque, G. G., H. J. Nauwynck, K. Van Reeth, and M. B. Pensaert. 2000. Effect of cellular changes and onset of humoral immunity on the replication of porcine reproductive & respiratory syndrome virus in the lungs of pigs. Journal of General Virology **81:** 1327-1334.

64. Lee, J. A., N. H. Lee, S. W. Lee, S. Y. Park, C. S. Song, I. S. Choi, and J. B. Lee. 2014. Development of a chimeric strain of porcine reproductive and respiratory syndrome virus with an infectious clone and a Korean dominant field strain. J Microbiol **52:** 345-349.

65. Lee, S. M., S. K. Schommer, and S. B. Kleiboeker. 2004. Porcine reproductive and respiratory syndrome virus field isolates differ in in-vitro interferon phenotypes. Vet Immunol Immunopathol **102:** 217-231.

66. Li, Z., G. Wang, Y. Wang, C. Zhang, B. Huang, Q. Li, L. Li, B. Xue, P. Ding, X. Cai, C. Wang, and E. M. Zhou. 2015. Immune responses of pigs immunized with a recombinant porcine reproductive and respiratory syndrome virus expressing porcine GM-CSF. Vet Immunol Immunopathol **168:** 40-48.

67. Li, Z., G. Wang, Y. Wang, C. Zhang, X. Wang, B. Huang, Q. Li, L. Li, B. Xue, P. Ding, S. F. Syed, C. Wang, X. Cai, and E. M. Zhou. 2015. Rescue and evaluation of a recombinant PRRSV expressing porcine Interleukin-4. Virol J **12:** 185.

68. Liu, C. H., H. C. Chaung, H. L. Chang, Y. T. Peng, and W. B. Chung. 2009. Expression of Toll-like receptor mRNA and cytokines in pigs infected with porcine reproductive and respiratory syndrome virus. Vet Microbiol **136:** 266-276.

69. Loemba, H. D., S. Mounir, H. Mardassi, D. Archambault, and S. Dea. 1996. Kinetics of humoral immune response to the major structural proteins of the porcine reproductive and respiratory syndrome virus. Arch Virol **141:** 751-761.

70. Lopez-Fuertes, L., E. Campos, N. Domenech, A. Ezquerra, J. M. Castro, J. Dominguez, and F. Alonso. 2000. Porcine reproductive and respiratory syndrome (PRRS) virus down-modulates TNF-alpha production in infected macrophages. Virus Res **69:** 41-46.

71. Lopez, O. J., M. F. Oliveira, E. A. Garcia, B. J. Kwon, A. Doster, and F. A. Osorio. 2007. Protection against porcine reproductive and respiratory syndrome virus (PRRSV) infection through passive transfer of PRRSV-neutralizing antibodies is dose dependent. Clinical and Vaccine Immunology **14:** 269-275.

72. Lopez, O. J., and F. A. Osorio. 2004. Role of neutralizing antibodies in PRRSV protective immunity. Vet Immunol Immunopathol **102:** 155-163.

73. Loving, C. L., F. A. Osorio, M. P. Murtaugh, and F. A. Zuckermann. 2015. Innate and adaptive immunity against Porcine Reproductive and Respiratory Syndrome Virus. Vet Immunol Immunopathol **167:** 1-14.

74. Lowe, J. E., R. Husmann, L. D. Firkins, F. A. Zuckermann, and T. L. Goldberg. 2005. Correlation of cell-mediated immunity against porcine reproductive and respiratory syndrome virus with protection against reproductive failure in sows during outbreaks of porcine reproductive and respiratory syndrome in commercial herds. J Am Vet Med Assoc **226:** 1707-1711.

75. Luo, R., S. Xiao, Y. Jiang, H. Jin, D. Wang, M. Liu, H. Chen, and L. Fang. 2008. Porcine reproductive and respiratory syndrome virus (PRRSV) suppresses interferon-beta production by interfering with the RIG-I signaling pathway. Mol Immunol **45:** 2839-2846.

76. Mair, K. H., H. Koinig, W. Gerner, A. Hohne, J. Bretthauer, J. J. Kroll, M. B. Roof, A. Saalmuller, K. Stadler, and R. Libanova. 2015. Carbopol improves the early cellular immune responses induced by the modified-life vaccine Ingelvac PRRS(R) MLV. Vet Microbiol **176:** 352-357.

77. Mardassi, H., B. Massie, and S. Dea. 1996. Intracellular synthesis, processing, and transport of proteins encoded by ORFs 5 to 7 of porcine reproductive and respiratory syndrome virus. Virology **221:** 98-112.

78. Martelli, P., S. Gozio, L. Ferrari, S. Rosina, E. De Angelis, C. Quintavalla, E. Bottarelli, and P. Borghetti. 2009. Efficacy of a modified live porcine reproductive and respiratory syndrome virus (PRRSV) vaccine in pigs naturally exposed to a heterologous European (Italian cluster) field strain: Clinical protection and cell-mediated immunity. Vaccine **27:** 3788-3799.

79. Mateu, E., and I. Diaz. 2008. The challenge of PRRS immunology. Vet J **177:** 345-351.

80. Meier, W. A., J. Galeota, F. A. Osorio, R. J. Husmann, W. M. Schnitzlein, and F. A. Zuckermann. 2003. Gradual development of the interferon-gamma response of swine to porcine reproductive and respiratory syndrome virus infection or vaccination. Virology **309:** 18-31.

81. Meier, W. A., R. J. Husmann, W. M. Schnitzlein, F. A. Osorio, J. K. Lunney, and F. A. Zuckermann. 2004. Cytokines and synthetic double-stranded RNA augment the T helper 1 immune response of swine to porcine reproductive and respiratory syndrome virus. Vet Immunol Immunopathol **102:** 299-314.

82. Meng, X. J. 2000. Heterogeneity of porcine reproductive and respiratory syndrome virus: implications for current vaccine efficacy and future vaccine development. Vet Microbiol **74:** 309-329.

83. Meng, X. J., P. S. Paul, P. G. Halbur, and M. A. Lum. 1995. Phylogenetic analyses of the putative M (ORF 6) and N (ORF 7) genes of porcine reproductive and respiratory syndrome virus (PRRSV): implication for the existence of two genotypes of PRRSV in the U.S.A. and Europe. Arch Virol **140:** 745-755.

84. Mengeling, W. L., K. M. Lager, A. C. Vorwald, and D. F. Clouser. 2003. Comparative safety and efficacy of attenuated single-strain and multi-strain vaccines for porcine reproductive and respiratory syndrome. Vet Microbiol **93:** 25-38.

85. Meulenberg, J. J., R. J. Bende, J. M. Pol, G. Wensvoort, and R. J. Moormann. 1995. Nucleocapsid protein N of Lelystad virus: expression by recombinant baculovirus, immunological properties, and suitability for detection of serum antibodies. Clin Diagn Lab Immunol **2:** 652-656.

86. Meulenberg, J. J., J. N. Bos-de Ruijter, G. Wensvoort, and R. J. Moormann. 1998. An infectious cDNA clone of porcine reproductive and respiratory syndrome virus. Adv Exp Med Biol **440:** 199-206.

87. Meulenberg, J. J., and A. Petersen-den Besten. 1996. Identification and characterization of a sixth structural protein of Lelystad virus: the glycoprotein GP2 encoded by ORF2 is incorporated in virus particles. Virology **225:** 44-51.

88. Meulenberg, J. J., A. P. van Nieuwstadt, A. van Essen-Zandbergen, and J. P. Langeveld. 1997. Post-translational processing and identification of a neutralization domain of the GP4 protein encoded by ORF4 of Lelystad virus. J Virol **71:** 6061-6067.

89. **Miguel, J. C., J. Chen, W. G. Van Alstine, and R. W. Johnson.** 2010. Expression of inflammatory cytokines and Toll-like receptors in the brain and respiratory tract of pigs infected with porcine reproductive and respiratory syndrome virus. Vet Immunol Immunopathol **135:** 314-319.

90. Mokhtar, H., L. Biffar, S. Somavarapu, J. P. Frossard, S. McGowan, M. Pedrera, R. Strong, J. C. Edwards, M. Garcia-Duran, M. J. Rodriguez, G. R. Stewart, F. Steinbach, and S. P. Graham. 2017. Evaluation of hydrophobic chitosan-based particulate formulations of porcine reproductive and respiratory syndrome virus vaccine candidate T cell antigens. Vet Microbiol.

91. Mulupuri, P., J. J. Zimmerman, J. Hermann, C. R. Johnson, J. P. Cano, W. Yu, S. A. Dee, and M. P. Murtaugh. 2008. Antigen-specific B-cell responses to porcine reproductive and respiratory syndrome virus infection. J Virol **82:** 358-370.

92. **Murtaugh, M. P., M. R. Elam, and L. T. Kakach.** 1995. Comparison of the structural protein coding sequences of the VR-2332 and Lelystad virus strains of the PRRS virus. Arch Virol **140:** 1451-1460.

93. **Murtaugh, M. P., and M. Genzow.** 2011. Immunological solutions for treatment and prevention of porcine reproductive and respiratory syndrome (PRRS). Vaccine **29:** 8192-8204.

94. **Murtaugh, M. P., T. Stadejek, J. E. Abrahante, T. T. Lam, and F. C. Leung.** 2010. The ever-expanding diversity of porcine reproductive and respiratory syndrome virus. Virus Res **154:** 18-30.

95. **Murtaugh, M. P., Z. Xiao, and F. Zuckermann.** 2002. Immunological responses of swine to porcine reproductive and respiratory syndrome virus infection. Viral Immunol **15:** 533-547.

96. **Nelsen, C. J., M. P. Murtaugh, and K. S. Faaberg.** 1999. Porcine reproductive and respiratory syndrome virus comparison: divergent evolution on two continents. J Virol **73:** 270-280.

97. **Nelson, E. A., J. Christopher-Hennings, and D. A. Benfield.** 1994. Serum immune responses to the proteins of porcine reproductive and respiratory syndrome (PRRS) virus. J Vet Diagn Invest **6:** 410-415.

98. **Nielsen, H. S., G. Liu, J. Nielsen, M. B. Oleksiewicz, A. Botner, T. Storgaard, and K. S. Faaberg.** 2003. Generation of an infectious clone of VR-2332, a highly virulent North American-type isolate of porcine reproductive and respiratory syndrome virus. J Virol **77:** 3702-3711.

99. **Nielsen, J., and A. Botner.** 1997. Hematological and immunological parameters of 4 1/2-month old pigs infected with PRRS virus. Vet Microbiol **55:** 289-294.

100. **Okuda, Y., M. Kuroda, M. Ono, S. Chikata, and I. Shibata.** 2008. Efficacy of vaccination with porcine reproductive and respiratory syndrome virus following challenges with field isolates in Japan. J Vet Med Sci **70:** 1017-1025.

101. **Oleksiewicz, M. B., A. Botner, P. Toft, P. Normann, and T. Storgaard.** 2001. Epitope mapping porcine reproductive and respiratory syndrome virus by phage display: the nsp2 fragment of the replicase polyprotein contains a cluster of B-cell epitopes. J Virol **75:** 3277-3290.

102. **Ostrowski, M., J. A. Galeota, A. M. Jar, K. B. Platt, F. A. Osorio, and O. J. Lopez.** 2002. Identification of neutralizing and nonneutralizing epitopes in the porcine reproductive and respiratory syndrome virus GP5 ectodomain. J Virol **76:** 4241-4250.

103. **Overend, C., R. Mitchell, D. He, G. Rompato, M. J. Grubman, and A. E. Garmendia.** 2007. Recombinant swine beta interferon protects swine alveolar macrophages and MARC-145 cells from infection with Porcine reproductive and respiratory syndrome virus. Journal of General Virology **88:** 925-931.

104. **Parida, R., I. S. Choi, D. A. Peterson, A. K. Pattnaik, W. Laegreid, F. A. Zuckermann, and F. A. Osorio.** 2012. Location of T-cell epitopes in non-structural proteins 9 and 10 of type-II porcine reproductive and respiratory syndrome virus. Virus Res **169:** 13-21.

105. **Park, J. Y., H. S. Kim, and S. H. Seo.** 2008. Characterization of interaction between porcine reproductive and respiratory syndrome

virus and porcine dendritic cells. J Microbiol Biotechnol **18:** 1709-1716.

106. **Peng, Y. T., H. C. Chaung, H. L. Chang, H. C. Chang, and W. B. Chung.** 2009. Modulations of phenotype and cytokine expression of porcine bone marrow-derived dendritic cells by porcine reproductive and respiratory syndrome virus. Vet Microbiol **136:** 359-365.

107. **Pirzadeh, B., and S. Dea.** 1998. Immune response in pigs vaccinated with plasmid DNA encoding ORF5 of porcine reproductive and respiratory syndrome virus. Journal of General Virology **79(Pt 5):** 989-999.

108. **Pirzadeh, B., and S. Dea.** 1997. Monoclonal antibodies to the ORF5 product of porcine reproductive and respiratory syndrome virus define linear neutralizing determinants. Journal of General Virology **78(Pt 8):** 1867-1873.

109. **Plagemann, P. G.** 2004. GP5 ectodomain epitope of porcine reproductive and respiratory syndrome virus, strain Lelystad virus. Virus Res **102:** 225-230.

110. **Plagemann, P. G.** 2006. Neutralizing antibody formation in swine infected with seven strains of porcine reproductive and respiratory syndrome virus as measured by indirect ELISA with peptides containing the GP5 neutralization epitope. Viral Immunol **19:** 285-293.

111. **Plagemann, P. G., R. R. Rowland, and K. S. Faaberg.** 2002. The primary neutralization epitope of porcine respiratory and reproductive syndrome virus strain VR-2332 is located in the middle of the GP5 ectodomain. Arch Virol **147:** 2327-2347.

112. **Plana Duran, J., I. Climent, J. Sarraseca, A. Urniza, E. Cortes, C. Vela, and J. I. Casal.** 1997. Baculovirus expression of proteins of porcine reproductive and respiratory syndrome virus strain Olot/91. Involvement of ORF3 and ORF5 proteins in protection. Virus Genes **14:** 19-29.

113. **Pujhari, S., T. T. Baig, and A. N. Zakhartchouk.** 2014. Potential role of porcine reproductive and respiratory syndrome virus structural protein GP2 in apoptosis inhibition. Biomed Res Int **2014:** 160505.

114. **Rodriguez-Gomez, I. M., T. Kaser, J. Gomez-Laguna, B. Lamp, L. Sinn, T. Rumenapf, L. Carrasco, A. Saalmuller, and W. Gerner.** 2015. PRRSV-infected monocyte-derived dendritic cells express high

levels of SLA-DR and CD80/86 but do not stimulate PRRSV-naive regulatory T cells to proliferate. Vet Res **46:** 54.

115. **Roques, E., A. Girard, M. C. St-Louis, B. Massie, C. A. Gagnon, M. Lessard, and D. Archambault.** 2013. Immunogenic and protective properties of GP5 and M structural proteins of porcine reproductive and respiratory syndrome virus expressed from replicating but non-disseminating adenovectors. Vet Res **44:** 17.

116. **Rowland, R. R., B. Robinson, J. Stefanick, T. S. Kim, L. Guanghua, S. R. Lawson, and D. A. Benfield.** 2001. Inhibition of porcine reproductive and respiratory syndrome virus by interferon-gamma and recovery of virus replication with 2-aminopurine. Arch Virol **146:** 539-555.

117. **Rowland, R. R., and D. Yoo.** 2003. Nucleolar-cytoplasmic shuttling of PRRSV nucleocapsid protein: a simple case of molecular mimicry or the complex regulation by nuclear import, nucleolar localization and nuclear export signal sequences. Virus Res **95:** 23-33.

118. **Sang, Y., R. R. Rowland, and F. Blecha.** 2014. Antiviral regulation in porcine monocytic cells at different activation states. J Virol **88:** 11395-11410.

119. **Sang, Y., J. Shi, W. Sang, R. R. Rowland, and F. Blecha.** 2012. Replication-competent recombinant porcine reproductive and respiratory syndrome (PRRS) viruses expressing indicator proteins and antiviral cytokines. Viruses **4:** 102-116.

120. **Scortti, M., C. Prieto, E. Alvarez, I. Simarro, and J. M. Castro.** 2007. Failure of an inactivated vaccine against porcine reproductive and respiratory syndrome to protect gilts against a heterologous challenge with PRRSV. Vet Rec **161:** 809-813.

121. **Shi, M., T. T. Lam, C. C. Hon, R. K. Hui, K. S. Faaberg, T. Wennblom, M. P. Murtaugh, T. Stadejek, and F. C. Leung.** 2010. Molecular epidemiology of PRRSV: a phylogenetic perspective. Virus Res **154:** 7-17.

122. **Shi, M., T. T. Lam, C. C. Hon, M. P. Murtaugh, P. R. Davies, R. K. Hui, J. Li, L. T. Wong, C. W. Yip, J. W. Jiang, and F. C. Leung.** 2010. Phylogeny-based evolutionary, demographical & geographical dissection of North American type 2 porcine reproductive and respiratory syndrome viruses. J Virol **84:** 8700-8711.

123. **Shi, M., T. T. Lam, C. C. Hon, M. P. Murtaugh, P. R. Davies, R. K. Hui, J. Li, L. T. Wong, C. W. Yip, J. W. Jiang, and F. C. Leung.** 2010. Phylogeny-based evolutionary, demographical and

geographical dissection of North American type 2 porcine reproductive and respiratory syndrome viruses. J Virol **84:** 8700-8711.

124. **Shimizu, M., S. Yamada, K. Kawashima, S. Ohashi, S. Shimizu, and T. Ogawa.** 1996. Changes of lymphocyte subpopulations in pigs infected with porcine reproductive and respiratory syndrome (PRRS) virus. Vet Immunol Immunopathol **50:** 19-27.

125. **Silva-Campa, E., L. Cordoba, L. Fraile, L. Flores-Mendoza, M. Montoya, and J. Hernandez.** 2010. European genotype of porcine reproductive and respiratory syndrome (PRRSV) infects monocyte-derived dendritic cells but does not induce Treg cells. Virology **396:** 264-271.

126. **Silva-Campa, E., L. Flores-Mendoza, M. Resendiz, A. Pinelli-Saavedra, V. Mata-Haro, W. Mwangi, and J. Hernandez.** 2009. Induction of T helper 3 regulatory cells by dendritic cells infected with porcine reproductive and respiratory syndrome virus. Virology **387:** 373-379.

127. **Silva-Campa, E., V. Mata-Haro, E. Mateu, and J. Hernandez.** 2012. Porcine reproductive and respiratory syndrome virus induces CD4+CD8+CD25+Foxp3+ regulatory T cells (Tregs). Virology **430:** 73-80.

128. **Song, S., J. Bi, D. Wang, L. Fang, L. Zhang, F. Li, H. Chen, and S. Xiao.** 2013. Porcine reproductive and respiratory syndrome virus infection activates IL-10 production through NF-kappaB and p38 MAPK pathways in porcine alveolar macrophages. Dev Comp Immunol **39:** 265-272.

129. **Stobart, C. C., and M. L. Moore.** 2014. RNA virus reverse genetics and vaccine design. Viruses **6:** 2531-2550.

130. **Sun, Y., M. Han, C. Kim, J. G. Calvert, and D. Yoo.** 2012. Interplay between interferon-mediated innate immunity and porcine reproductive and respiratory syndrome virus. Viruses **4:** 424-446.

131. **Sur, J. H., A. R. Doster, and F. A. Osorio.** 1998. Apoptosis induced in vivo during acute infection by porcine reproductive and respiratory syndrome virus. Vet Pathol **35:** 506-514.

132. **Suradhat, S., S. Kesdangsakonwut, W. Sada, S. Buranapraditkun, S. Wongsawang, and R. Thanawongnuwech.** 2006. Negative impact of porcine reproductive and respiratory syndrome virus infection on the efficacy of classical swine fever vaccine. Vaccine **24:** 2634-2642.

133. **Takikawa, N., S. Kobayashi, S. Ide, Y. Yamane, Y. Tanaka, and H. Yamagishi.** 1996. Detection of antibodies against porcine reproductive and respiratory syndrome (PRRS) virus in swine sera by enzyme-linked immunosorbent assay. J Vet Med Sci **58:** 355-357.

134. **Thaa, B., B. C. Sinhadri, C. Tielesch, E. Krause, and M. Veit.** 2013. Signal peptide cleavage from GP5 of PRRSV: a minor fraction of molecules retains the decoy epitope, a presumed molecular cause for viral persistence. PLoS One **8:** e65548.

135. **Thanawongnuwech, R., T. F. Young, B. J. Thacker, and E. L. Thacker.** 2001. Differential production of proinflammatory cytokines: in-vitro PRRSV and Mycoplasma hyopneumoniae co-infection model. Vet Immunol Immunopathol **79:** 115-127.

136. **Tian, D., Z. Wei, J. C. Zevenhoven-Dobbe, R. Liu, G. Tong, E. J. Snijder, and S. Yuan.** 2012. Arterivirus minor envelope proteins are a major determinant of viral tropism in cell culture. J Virol **86:** 3701-3712.

137. **Trible, B. R., L. N. Popescu, N. Monday, J. G. Calvert, and R. R. Rowland.** 2015. A single amino acid deletion in the matrix protein of porcine reproductive and respiratory syndrome virus confers resistance to a polyclonal swine antibody with broadly neutralizing activity. J Virol **89:** 6515-6520.

138. **Truong, H. M., Z. Lu, G. F. Kutish, J. Galeota, F. A. Osorio, and A. K. Pattnaik.** 2004. A highly pathogenic porcine reproductive and respiratory syndrome virus generated from an infectious cDNA clone retains the in-vivo virulence and transmissibility properties of the parental virus. Virology **325:** 308-319.

139. **Van Gorp, H., W. Van Breedam, P. L. Delputte, and H. J. Nauwynck.** 2008. Sialoadhesin and CD163 join forces during entry of the porcine reproductive and respiratory syndrome virus. Journal of General Virology **89:** 2943-2953.

140. **van Gucht, S., K. van Reeth, and M. Pensaert.** 2003. Interaction between porcine reproductive-respiratory syndrome virus and bacterial endotoxin in the lungs of pigs: potentiation of cytokine production and respiratory disease. J Clin Microbiol **41:** 960-966.

141. **van Nieuwstadt, A. P., J. J. Meulenberg, A. van Essen-Zanbergen, A. Petersen-den Besten, R. J. Bende, R. J. Moormann, and G. Wensvoort.** 1996. Proteins encoded by open reading frames 3 and 4 of the genome of Lelystad virus (Arteriviridae) are structural proteins of the virion. J Virol **70:** 4767-4772.

142. **Van Reeth, K., G. Labarque, H. Nauwynck, and M. Pensaert.** 1999. Differential production of proinflammatory cytokines in the pig lung during different respiratory virus infections: correlations with pathogenicity. Res Vet Sci **67:** 47-52.

143. **Vanderheijden, N., P. L. Delputte, H. W. Favoreel, J. Vandekerckhove, J. Van Damme, P. A. van Woensel, and H. J. Nauwynck.** 2003. Involvement of sialoadhesin in entry of porcine reproductive and respiratory syndrome virus into porcine alveolar macrophages. J Virol **77:** 8207-8215.

144. **Vanhee, M., P. L. Delputte, I. Delrue, M. F. Geldhof, and H. J. Nauwynck.** 2009. Development of an experimental inactivated PRRSV vaccine that induces virus-neutralizing antibodies. Vet Res **40:** 63.

145. **Vanhee, M., W. Van Breedam, S. Costers, M. Geldhof, Y. Noppe, and H. Nauwynck.** 2011. Characterization of antigenic regions in the porcine reproductive and respiratory syndrome virus by the use of peptide-specific serum antibodies. Vaccine **29:** 4794-4804.

146. **Vashisht, K., K. R. Erlandson, L. D. Firkins, F. A. Zuckermann, and T. L. Goldberg.** 2008. Evaluation of contact exposure as a method for acclimatizing growing pigs to porcine reproductive and respiratory syndrome virus. J Am Vet Med Assoc **232:** 1530-1535.

147. **Vu, H. L., B. Kwon, K. J. Yoon, W. W. Laegreid, A. K. Pattnaik, and F. A. Osorio.** 2011. Immune evasion of porcine reproductive and respiratory syndrome virus through glycan shielding involves both glycoprotein 5 as well as glycoprotein 3. J Virol **85:** 5555-5564.

148. **Vu, H. L., B. Kwon, K. J. Yoon, W. W. Laegreid, A. K. Pattnaik, and F. A. Osorio.** 2011. Immune evasion of porcine reproductive and respiratory syndrome virus through glycan shielding involves both glycoprotein 5 as well as glycoprotein 3. J Virol **85:** 5555-5564.

149. **Wang, G., T. Song, Y. Yu, Y. Liu, W. Shi, S. Wang, F. Rong, J. Dong, H. Liu, X. Cai, and E. M. Zhou.** 2011. Immune responses in piglets infected with highly pathogenic porcine reproductive and respiratory syndrome virus. Vet Immunol Immunopathol **142:** 170-178.

150. **Weiland, E., M. Wieczorek-Krohmer, D. Kohl, K. K. Conzelmann, and F. Weiland.** 1999. Monoclonal antibodies to the GP5 of porcine reproductive and respiratory syndrome virus are more effective in virus neutralization than monoclonal antibodies to the GP4. Vet Microbiol **66:** 171-186.

151. **Welch, S. K., R. Jolie, D. S. Pearce, W. D. Koertje, E. Fuog, S. L. Shields, D. Yoo, and J. G. Calvert.** 2004. Construction and evaluation of genetically engineered replication-defective porcine reproductive and respiratory syndrome virus vaccine candidates. Vet Immunol Immunopathol **102:** 277-290.

152. **Wieringa, R., A. A. de Vries, and P. J. Rottier.** 2003. Formation of disulfide-linked complexes between the three minor envelope glycoproteins (GP2b, GP3, and GP4) of equine arteritis virus. J Virol **77:** 6216-6226.

153. **Wissink, E. H., M. V. Kroese, H. A. van Wijk, F. A. Rijsewijk, J. J. Meulenberg, and P. J. Rottier.** 2005. Envelope protein requirements for the assembly of infectious virions of porcine reproductive and respiratory syndrome virus. J Virol **79:** 12495-12506.

154. **Wongyanin, P., S. Buranapraditkun, K. Chokeshai-Usaha, R. Thanawonguwech, and S. Suradhat.** 2010. Induction of inducible CD4+CD25+Foxp3+ regulatory T lymphocytes by porcine reproductive and respiratory syndrome virus (PRRSV). Vet Immunol Immunopathol **133:** 170-182.

155. **Wu, W. H., Y. Fang, R. Farwell, M. Steffen-Bien, R. R. Rowland, J. Christopher-Hennings, and E. A. Nelson.** 2001. A 10-kDa structural protein of porcine reproductive and respiratory syndrome virus encoded by ORF2b. Virology **287:** 183-191.

156. **Xiao, Z., C. A. Trincado, and M. P. Murtaugh.** 2004. Beta-glucan enhancement of T cell IFNgamma response in swine. Vet Immunol Immunopathol **102:** 315-320.

157. **Yang, L., M. L. Frey, K. J. Yoon, J. J. Zimmerman, and K. B. Platt.** 2000. Categorization of North American porcine reproductive and respiratory syndrome viruses: epitopic profiles of the N, M, GP5 and GP3 proteins and susceptibility to neutralization. Arch Virol **145:** 1599-1619.

158. **Yoo, D., S. K. Welch, C. Lee, and J. G. Calvert.** 2004. Infectious cDNA clones of porcine reproductive and respiratory syndrome virus and their potential as vaccine vectors. Vet Immunol Immunopathol **102:** 143-154.

159. **Yoon, I. J., H. S. Joo, S. M. Goyal, and T. W. Molitor.** 1994. A modified serum neutralization test for the detection of antibody to porcine reproductive and respiratory syndrome virus in swine sera. J Vet Diagn Invest **6:** 289-292.

160. **Yoon, K. J., L. L. Wu, J. J. Zimmerman, H. T. Hill, and K. B. Platt.** 1996. Antibody-dependent enhancement (ADE) of porcine reproductive and respiratory syndrome virus (PRRSV) infection in pigs. Viral Immunol **9:** 51-63.

161. **Yoon, K. J., L. L. Wu, J. J. Zimmerman, and K. B. Platt.** 1997. Field isolates of porcine reproductive and respiratory syndrome virus (PRRSV) vary in their susceptibility to antibody dependent enhancement (ADE) of infection. Vet Microbiol **55:** 277-287.

162. **Yu, D., J. Lv, Z. Sun, H. Zheng, J. Lu, and S. Yuan.** 2009. Reverse genetic manipulation of the overlapping coding regions for structural proteins of the type II porcine reproductive and respiratory syndrome virus. Virology **383:** 22-31.

163. **Yuan, S., and Z. Wei.** 2008. Construction of infectious cDNA clones of PRRSV: separation of coding regions for non-structural and structural proteins. Sci China C Life Sci **51:** 271-279.

164. **Zhou, L., Y. Y. Ni, P. Pineyro, C. M. Cossaboom, S. Subramaniam, B. J. Sanford, B. A. Dryman, Y. W. Huang, and X. J. Meng.** 2013. Broadening the heterologous cross-neutralizing antibody inducing ability of porcine reproductive and respiratory syndrome virus by breeding the GP4 or M genes. PLoS One **8:** e66645.

165. **Zhou, L., Y. Y. Ni, P. Pineyro, B. J. Sanford, C. M. Cossaboom, B. A. Dryman, Y. W. Huang, D. J. Cao, and X. J. Meng.** 2012. DNA shuffling of the GP3 genes of porcine reproductive and respiratory syndrome virus (PRRSV) produces a chimeric virus with an improved cross-neutralizing ability against a heterologous PRRSV strain. Virology **434:** 96-109.

166. **Zuckermann, F. A., E. A. Garcia, I. D. Luque, J. Christopher-Hennings, A. Doster, M. Brito, and F. Osorio.** 2007. Assessment of the efficacy of commercial porcine reproductive and respiratory syndrome virus (PRRSV) vaccines based on measurement of serologic response, frequency of gamma-IFN-producing cells and virological parameters of protection upon challenge. Vet Microbiol **123:** 69-85.

167. **Zuckermann, F. A., and R. J. Husmann.** 1996. Functional and phenotypic analysis of porcine peripheral blood CD4/CD8 double-positive T cells. Immunology **87:** 500-512.

4

Livestock Based Integrated Farming Systems for Resource Conservation and Sustainability

Ravindra Kumar*, Sushil Prasad and Dhirendra Kumar

* Department of Livestock Production & Management, Ranchi Veterinary College, BAU, Ranchi

Indian agriculture can largely be characterized as rain fed small holders' production system, with a special significance to livestock in attaining sustainability, hedging risk and creation of livelihood. The share of livestock for under-privileged marginal and landless livestock owner is as high as 70-80% during drought year. There is substantial deficit in forage availability in almost all parts of the country. Forage based feeding system under the crop livestock integrated farming system and under intensive dairy production will ensure reduced cost of production leading to livelihood improvement and profitability. Under such scenario, there is need for IFS approach in agricultural production system for sustainability, employment, profitability, resource use efficiency and health. FAO (1977) stated that "there is no waste", and "waste is only a misplaced resource which can become a valuable material for another product" in IFS. The integrated farming systems approach holds the key for socio-economic upliftment of rural households as it judiciously combines crop, trees, livestock, fishery, etc. in a holistic manner and has the potential to meet the diverse needs of the farming communities on sustainable basis. IFS activity is focused around a few selected interdependent, inter-related and interlinking production system based on crops, animals and related subsidiary professions. The growth rate of agriculture in the recent past is very slow in spite of the rapid economic growth in India. According to the Economic Survey of India, 2008, the growth rate of food grain production decelerated to 1.2% during 1990-2007, lower than the population growth of 1.9%. It is projected that in our country population will touch 1370 million by 2030 and to 1600 million by 2050. To meet the demand, we have to produce 289 and 349 mt of food grains during the respective periods. The current scenario in the country indicates that area under cultivation may further dwindle and more than 20% of current cultivable area will be converted for non-agricultural purposes by 2030 (Gill *et al.*, 2005). Practically there is no scope for horizontal expansion of land for agriculture, only vertical expansion is possible by integrating farming components requiring lesser space and time and ensuring reasonable returns to farm families. Thus, Integrated farming system approach is not only a reliable way of obtaining fairly high productivity with considerable scope for resource recycling, but also concept of ecological soundness leading to sustainable agriculture.

Elements of Integrated Farming System

Elements may be included in IFS demonstrations depending upon the individual farmers resources, interest and opportunities. These are watershed, farm ponds, bio-pesticides, bio-fertilizers, plant products as pesticides, bio-gas, solar energy, compost making (Vermi, Japanese, Improved, etc.), green manuring, rainwater harvesting, etc.

Scope of farming system

A combination of one or more livestock enterprises with cropping, when carefully chosen, planned and executed, gives greater dividends than a single enterprise, especially for small and marginal farmers. Farm as a unit is to be considered and planned for effective integration of the enterprises to be combined with crop production activity. Integration of farm enterprises to be combined on many factors, such as:

- Soil and climatic features of the selected area.
- Availability of resources, land, labour and capital.
- Present level of utilization of resources.
- Economics of proposed integrated farming system.
- Managerial skill of the farmer.

Goals of Integrated Farming System

The four primary goals of IFS are:

i) Maximization of yield of all component enterprises to provide steady and stable income.

ii) Rejuvenation / amelioration of system's productivity and achieve agro-ecological equilibrium.

iii) Avoid build-up of insect-pests, diseases and weed population through natural cropping system management and keep them at low level of intensity.

iv) Reducing the use of chemicals (fertilizers and pesticides) to provide chemical free healthy produce and environment to the society.

Choice of Enterprise

Livestock is the best complimentary enterprise with cropping. Installation of bio-digester in crop-livestock system will make use of the wastes, at the same time provides valuable gas for cooking and lighting.

Components in IFS

The components of IFS include crops, fish farming, poultry, pigs, cattle, sheep and goat, fodder production, kitchen gardening. Thamizoli *et al.* (2006) found that the introduction of tree crops with agriculture along with the farm based allied enterprises like dairy, goat rearing, apiculture, etc. as a risk management strategy to cope up with disasters like long drought season and heavy flood. Mohanty *et al.* (2010) identified the IFS model consists of field crops (Rice, groundnut, maize, pigeon, pea and ragi), horticultural crops (Yam, banana, tapioca and vegetables), vermin-composting and poultry (Vanaraja breed) in Gajapati district of Odisha. Tripathi and Rathi (2011) stated that various prevailing farming system models in Uttarakhand namely., crop + dairy, crop + dairy + goats + horticulture, crop + horticulture +goats, crop +dairy + vegetables, horticulture + dairy + vegetables, vegetables + dairy and crop + dairy + companion animals are the major components in IFS. Manivannan *et al.* (2011) reported that the respondents from Erode district of Tamilnadu were having goat +crop, goat +dairy + crop, goat + dairy and goat +dairy +crop systems as the main components in IFS. Vision 2030 (2011d) suggested that the integration of mono – crop agriculture with agro forestry, pisciculture and animal husbandry as an important components for resource utilization, enhancing farm income and livelihood security of farmers.

Economic Importance of ifs

Jayanthi *et al.* (2003) and Ravishankar *et al.* (2007) reported the findings of net returns obtained from all the components was Rs. 22,887 with an increase of 32.3 per cent higher returns than the conventional rice-rice system. Ramrao *et al.* (2005) developed a crop-livestock mixed farming model of 1.5 acre small scale holders with the employment generation of 571 man days, net income of Rs. 58,456 per year against crop farming alone with employment generation of 385 man days and net returns of Rs. 18,300 per year only. Ramrao *et al.* (2006) noticed that the mixed farming of 2 bullocks+ 1 cow+ 1buffalo + 10 goats+ 10 poultry and 10 ducks gave a net rreturn of Rs 33,076 compared to Rs 7843 from arable farming.

Benefits of livestock based integrated farming system

- Productivity improvement
- Net profit growth and fixed income
- Sustainable growth in agriculture
- Balanced diet pollution free environment
- Recycling of farm residues
- Increase in employment
- High standard of living

Constraints

Banerjee *et al.* (1990) revealed that the limited amount of capital as the main constraint in IFS. Ngambeki *et al.* (1992) revealed that the lack of animal feed throughout the year and unavailability of labour in needy times are the major production constraints in IFS. Thamrongwarangkul (2001) reported that resource-poor farmers are not able to invest more capital as initial investment as a constraint since there is need of immediate economic returns to meet their food requirements, schools, medical treatments and loan- repayment. Nageswaran *et al.* (2009) identified the constraints as of procuring the improved breeds of livestock, timely availability of fish seed and feed, low cost energy efficient pumping machine, information on government schemes and credit support from financial institutions. Kadam *et al.* (2010) observed that the constraints of IFS as high cost of concentrate feed and unavailability of green fodder (40 per cent) and 30 per cent of the respondents expressed lack of market facilities and absence of co-operative societies. Nutritional values of crop residues are generally low in digestibility and protein content. Improving intake and digestibility of crop residues by physical and chemical treatments is technically possible but not feasible for poor small farmers because they require machinery and chemicals that are expensive or not readily available (*Keftasa and International Livestock Centre for Africa, 1988*).

Challenges

- Develop strategies and promote crop livestock synergies and interactions that aim to:
  - a) Integrate crops and livestock effectively with careful land use;
  - b) Raise the productivity of specific mixed crop-livestock systems;
  - c) Facilitate expansion of food production; and
  - d) Simultaneously safeguard the environment with prudent and efficient use of natural resources.
- Devise measures (for instance, facilitating large scale dissemination of bio-digesters) to implement a more efficient use of biomass, reducing pressures on natural resources; and develop a sustainable livestock manure management system to control environmental losses and contaminant spreading. (Gupta *et. al.*, 2012).

Opportunities

- Intensification of agriculture which is currently occurring in most farming systems favours crop– livestock integration.
- Poor soil fertility, unavailability or increases in prices of fertilizers, and labour shortages, have forced farmers to rely on alternatives, such as manure and traction.
- Farmers can grow crop in the wet season and engage in livestock enterprises in the dry season.
- Livestock enterprises are more lucrative than crop farming, so it is advantageous to integrate livestock into farm activities.
- Many indigenous, emerging, and developed technologies are available to support sustainable crop–livestock integration. These include improved cereal and grain legume varieties, cropping systems, weed and nutrient management strategies, the eradication of most livestock diseases, and the development of modeling and all-year-round feed packages for animals.

Conclusion

Thus, it can be concluded that IFS with cropping involving poultry, fish and goat was highly productive and profitable. It can be advocated for small and medium farmers in middle and tail end of canal where waters is limiting. IFS can provide progressive economic growth, employment opportunities, family nutritional requirements, optimal utilization of resources of the farming enterprises, etc. Further need based integrated farming system models may be developed by researchers depending on the situation of area along with status and liking of farmers existing in the country and should be documented properly to reach the mass farmers. Although the integrated farming system has certain constraints the scientific community and research station has to initiate steps to alleviate such problems of the farmers to improve their standard of living and income.

References

1. Banerjee, B.N., Sarker S.C. and Maity A.K. (1990). Impact of resource optimization on cropping pattern and income on crop-dairy mixed farm. Indian Journal of Dairy Science, **43:** 295-301.
2. Biswas, B.C. (2010). Farming System Approach to Improve IUE, Employment and Income in Eastern India. Fertiliser Marketing News **41(5):** 6-12.
3. FAO. (1977). China. Recycling of organic wastes in agriculture. FAO Soil Bull., 40-Rome.
4. Jayanthi, C., Baluswamy, M., Chinnusamy, C. and Mythily, S. (2003). Integrated nutrient supply system of linked components in lowland integrated farming system. Indian Journal of Agronomy, **48:** 241- 246
5. Kadam, S.S., Hatey, A.A., Nikam, T.R., Landge, S.P., and Palampalley, H.Y. (2010). Constraints of IFS in Kankan region of Maharashtra - A case study. In: 22nd national seminar on "Role of Extension in Integrated Farming Systems for sustainable rural livelihood, 9th -10th Dec, Maharashtra, pp. 101.
6. Manivannan, A., Mathialagan, P. and Narmatha, N. (2011). Goat based farming system in Tamilnadu, pp. 163.
7. Mohanty, D., Patnaik, S.C., Jeevan Das, P., Parida, N.K. and Nedunchezhiyan, M. (2010). Sustainable livelihood: a success story of a tribal farmer. Odisha Review, September: 41-43.
8. Nageswaran, M., Selvaganapathy, E., Subbiah, V.R. and Nair, S. (2009). Demonstration and Replication of Integrated Farming Systems at Chidambaram. Report of M.S. Swaminathan Research Foundation (MSSRF), Chennai, pp. 16-53.
9. Ngambeki, D.S., Deuson, R.R. and Preckel, P.V. (1992). Integrating livestock into farming systems in northern Cameroon. Agricultural Systems, **38:** 319-338.

10. Ramrao, W.Y., Tiwari, S.P and Singh, P. (2006). Crop-livestock integrated farming system for the Marginal farmers in rain fed regions of Chhattisgarh in Central India. Livestock Research for Rural Development, **18(7)**.

11. Ramrao, W.Y., Tiwari, S.P. and Singh, P. (2005). Crop-livestock integrated farming system for augmenting socio-economic status of smallholder tribal of Chhattisgarh in central India. Livestock Research for Rural development, **17(90)**.

12. Ravishankar, N., Pramanik, S.C., Rai Shakila Nawaz, R.B., Tapan K.R., Biswas. and Nabisat, B. (2007). Study on integrated farming system in hilly upland areas of Bay Islands. Indian Journal of Agronomy, **52:** 7-10.

13. Thamizoli, P.R., Rengalakshmi, K., Senthilkumar. and Selvaraju, T. (2006). Agronomic Rehabilitation and Livelihood Restoration of Tsunami Affected Lands in Nagapattinam District of Tamilnadu. M.S. Swaminathan Research Foundation Chennai, pp. 31.

14. Thamrongwarangkul, A. (2001). For out Thailand. Annual report on sustainable community development for good livelihoods and environmental project. Khon Kaen University.

15. Tripathi, S.C. and Rathi, R.C. (2011). Livestock farming system module for hills. In: Souvenir. National symposium on technological interventions for sustainable agriculture, 3rd - 5th May, GBPUAT, hill campus, Ranichuri, pp. 103-104.

16. Vision 2030. (2011d). Central Soil Salinity Research Institute (CSSRI), Karnal, pp. 15.

17. Vinod Gupta., Rai, P.K. and Risam K.S. (2012) Indian Research Journal of Extension Education, Special Issue (Volume II), 2012.

18. Manjunatha S.B., Shivmurthy D., Sunil, A.S., Nagaraj M.V., and Basavesha K.N. (2014). Integrated Farming System - An Holistic Approach: A Review Research and Reviews: Journal of Agriculture and Allied Sciences.

19. Gill M.S., Samra, J.S. and Singh, Gurbachan. (2005). Integrated farming system for realizing high productivity under shallow water-table conditions. Research bulletins, Department of Agronomy, PAU, Ludhiana, pp. 1-29.

❑❑❑

5

Global Warming Mitigation Through Improved Livestock Management

Ravindra Kumar* and Dhirendra Kumar

*Department of Livestock Production & Management, Ranchi Veterinary College, BAU, Ranchi

Global warming is an international problem. The major gases having greenhouse effect in the atmosphere CO_2, CH_4, N_2O and hlorofluorocarbons. India ranks 5th in CO_2 plus CH_4 pollution and 2nd in methane gas pollution. Methane appears to be the major cause for global warming. Ruminant animals in this process of digestion, methane—a potential greenhouse gas—are produced as a product of enteric fermentation. Among the volatile fatty acids (VFAs) produced during the fermentation, acetate and butyrate are methanogenic and spare hydrogen during formation. Hydrogen produced is then utilized by the methanogenic microbes (archaebacteria) in the production of methane and later belched out of the animal's mouth and nose, or it can convert the acetic acid into methane. About 8 to 9 per cent of gross energy (GE) is lost as a result of methane production. Similarly, it was found that milk production level also affects the production of methane. Globally, ruminant livestock produce about 80 million metric tons of methane annually. In the total methane efflux the livestock contribute about 18 per cent and Indian livestock share is 13.2 per cent of total contribution of livestock (World Resources Institute, 1990). Methane has 23 times the global warming potential of $CO\text{-}_2$ and is expected to cause between 15 to 17 per cent of the global warming over the next 50 years. The meat industry is the largest emitter of methane among the various livestock industries as beef animals are often reared on poor quality feed with less-than-optimal management conditions. India, for example, with the largest livestock population at about 464 million (including the highest buffalo population) is greatly contributing to the global warming effects due to methane emission from livestock. Indian livestock produces approximately 8,995 Tg methane per year, or 405.75X108 Kcal per day. Global warming can cause alteration in living style of people due to following changes:

- Increase in earth's temperature.
- Melting of ice on the mountains, Arctic and Antarctic areas.
- Due to melting of ice and expansion of water, there is a rise in global sea level.
- Changes in ecosystem due to changed temperature and water availability in a particular area.
- Changes in pathogenesis of plants, animal and human beings.

Microbial Synthesis of Methane in the Rumen

Methanogenesis is carried out by a specialised group of micro-organisms (Methanobrevibacter and Methanomicrobium) that are not true bacteria (Miller, 1995). Rumen methanogens preferably synthesise methane from H_2 and CO_2 to generate their energy requirements for growth (Miller 1995) according to the reaction:

$$4H_2 + CO_2 = CH_4 + 2H_2O$$

The type of carbohydrate in the diet has an effect on methanogenesis. High starch-containing diets lower rumen pH, and methanogens are inhibited at low pH (Van Nevel & Demeyer, 1996). Conversely, high fibre diets tend to produce a high acetate/propionate ratio and increased methane.

Methane emission from the degradation of faeces (manure)

Undigested feed residues are voided via the faeces. Methane will be emitted from these faeces in three ways: release of trapped methane originating from gastro-intestinal digestion; some residual digestion by intestinal microbes and a slow subsequent release due to invasion by soil methanogenic archaea (Williams, 1993).

Factors Affecting Methane Emission

- **Feed intake :** The relationship between methane emission (g/d) and DM intake is positive, but characterised by high variability between animals (Kirchgessner *et al.*, 1995; Lassey *et al.*, 1997). This suggests that for efficient animal production and reduced methane emission it is advantageous to feed animals well above maintenance intake.

- **Diet composition :** The major constituents of the diet - sugars, starch, fibre, protein and lipid-appear to have varying impacts on methane emission. On average crude fibre provides about 60%, nitrogen-free extract 30%, crude protein 10% and ether extract a minor proportion of total methane production, (Kirchgessner *et al.*, 1995). Increasing protein and lipids in a diet would be expected to decrease methane emission (Dohme *et al.*, 1999).
- **Digestibility :** When feed is given at low levels of intake, methane emission increases as digestibility increases, whereas with high intakes methane emission falls as digestibility increases (Blaxter and Clapperton, 1965).

Relationship between Digestibility and Methane Emission at Different Levels of Feeding

Other factors

A number of other nutritional and physiological factors are known to influence methane emission, such as grinding and pelleting the diet, and frequency of feeding (Johnson & Johnson, 1995; Mathison *et al.*, 1998), but are probably of little significance under grazing.

MITIGATION OPTIONS

A wide range of possibilities for reducing the methane emission of grazing livestock has been suggested. These include reducing livestock numbers, increasing the efficiency of animal production, genetic improvement, antimethanogenic feed additives, immunisation, manipulation of the rumen microbial ecosystem and manipulation of farm management. These are the participating agencies engaged in reducing the methane production in India:

- Appropriate Technology India (ATI), Ahmedabad, Gujarat.
- National Dairy Development Board (NDDB) and District Dairy Co-operative Union in Gujarat, Anand, Gujarat.
- National Dairy Research Institute (NDRI), Karnal.

- Bharatiya Agro Industrial Foundation (BAIF), Development Research Foundation, Baroda, Gujarat.
- Self Employed Women's Association (SEWA), Ahmedabad, Gujarat.

Reduction in livestock numbers : As emissions from livestock is the predominant source of methane in countries like India. India ranks 1st in cattle and buffalo population and 70-75% of total population are non-descript or low producing. Livestock numbers are the major determinant of methane emission from pastoral agriculture, and it is implicit that reducing numbers is the simplest way to reduce emission.

Increasing the efficiency of livestock production : The higher the intake above maintenance, or the higher the level of production, the lower will be the methane emitted per unit of product and thus, the higher the efficiency with respect to methane.

Increasing feed intake : Increasing feed intake decreases the methane emission per unit of feed intake. This can also be seen in terms of production: as milk production (Kirchgessner *et al.*, 1995) increases an asymptotic decrease in methane emission per unit of product occurs. As intake increases, the proportion of the methane associated with maintenance declines. This is known as the dilution of maintenance as intake increases.

Table 1: Proportion of the Methane Emission Attributable to Maintenance or Milk Production in 450 kg Grazing Dairy Cows (Kirchgessner *et al.*, 1995)

DDMI	Milk yield	CH_4	% CH_4 associated with:		CH_4/milk
(kg/d)[1]	(kg/d)	(g/d)[2]	Maintenance	Production	(g/kg)
4.0	0	105	100	0	
7.9	12	206	51	49	17.2
10.5	20	272	39	61	13.6
11.7	24	305	34	66	12.7

Dietary manipulation : The type of diet fed to animals can have a major effect on methane production. Decreasing dietary fibre and increasing starch and lipid will reduce methane emission. Generally, diets of higher digestibility have these characteristics. This effect can be seen in the calculation in Table 2, where dairy cows were given feeds of increasing digestibility to achieve the same level of milk production.

Table 2: Effect of Feed Quality on Methane Emission of Cows at the Same Level of Milk Production (Benchar *et al.*, 2001)

DM digestibility (%)	55	65	75
Milk production (kg/d)	20	20	20
Feed intake (kg DM/d)	21.6	17.5	14.6
CH_4 emission (g/d) [1]	309	296	285
g CH_4/kg milk	15.5	14.8	14.3

Methane production (MJ/100MJ) could be reduced by increasing feed intake (-7%), increasing the concentrate proportion of the diet (-40%), replacing fibrous concentrate with starchy concentrate (-22%), with the utilisation of less ruminally degradable starch (-17%), increasing the digestibility of forage (-15%), with legume compared to grass forage (-28%) and with silage compared to hay (-20%). Feeding of total mixed ration, high quality leguminous forages, the addition of lipids (especially unsaturated fatty acids), alkali/ammonia treatment and grinding and pelleting of forages also help reduce methane emission. (Johnson & Johnson, 1995; Mathison *et al.*, 1998). The protection of protein by various techniques (treatment with heat, formaldehyde and tannic acid) produced a significant improvement in productivity and caused depression in methane production due to increased efficiency of fermentation, digestion and faster growth.

Metabolic efficiency : Treatment of animals with growth promoting substances like somatotrophin can result in increased efficiency of production (Bauman *et al.*, 1985). Thus, milk production per unit intake (efficiency) increased and methane emitted per kg milk was calculated to decrease.

Genetic improvement in animals to reduce methane emission : There are two aspects of genetic improvement with respect to methane emission genetic improvement in the efficiency of food conversion by the animals themselves; and the possibility that there are genetic differences between animals in the amount of methane they emit at the same feed intake. (Waghorn *et al.*, 2002)

Table 3: Methane Emission (g/kg DMI) from Dairy Cows of Two Genotypes Fed Two Different Diets. TMR = Total mixed rations. (Waghorn *et al.*, 2002)

	Days of lactation		
	60	**150**	**240**
Pasture diet:			
NZ genotype	18.0	22.2	23.8
US genotype	15.1	19.9	23.4
TMR diet:			
NZ genotype	20.2	22.0	22.3
US genotype	16.0	19.5	21.4

FEED ADDITIVES

A wide range of chemicals are available that will reduce rumen methanogenesis (Chalupa, 1980; Mathison et al, 1998). These are:

Alternative hydrogen acceptors : Sulphate/sulphite, dicarboxylic organic acids, malate, fumarate and nitrate/nitrite are potential alternative hydrogen acceptors. Addition of unsaturated fatty acids to the rumen will decrease methane emission. Their effect is twofold: the unsaturated fatty acids are a potential alternative sink for hydrogen, and large doses are toxic to rumen micro-organisms and depress digestion (*Krause 2002*).

Halogenated methane analogues : Many halogenated methane analogues such as chloroform, carbon tetrachloride, chloral hydrate, bromochloromethane and bromoethanesulphonic acid can be very potent methane inhibitors (*Mathison et al., 1998*).

Antibiotics : The effects of a wide range of antibiotics, including the ionophores, on methane production have been reviewed by *van Nevel and Demeyer (1995, 1996*) and *Johnson and Johnson* (*2002*). These antibiotics shift VFA patterns towards higher propionate, inhibit the growth of rumen methanogens.

Defaunating agents : Defaunation results in reductions in emission of about 20-50%. Defaunating agents, such as manoxol, teric, alkanate 3SL3 and sulphosuccinate act by disrupting the close symbiotic relationship between methanogenic bacteria and protozoa (*Mathison et al, 1998*).

Probiotics : There are mixed reports as to whether these probiotic (microbial feed additives) can reduce methane emission (*van Nevel & Demeyer, 1995; Moss et al., 2000*).

Bacteriocins : *Callaway et al. (1997)* used the bacteriocin nisin, which is produced by *Lactococcus lactis*, to produce a 36% reduction of methane production *in-vitro*.

Naturally ocurring plant compounds : There are naturally occurring compounds in some forages that appear to have antimethanogenic properties may be due to having condenced tannin or unidentified growth factor. eg. leaves of the tropical plant *Enterolobium timbouva* (*Gupta et al., 1993*), legume *Lotus corniculatus* (*Woodward et al. 2001*). Yucca extracts, fruit of Sapindus saponaria, methanol extracts of Sapindus rarak fruit.

Immunisation : Scientists in Australia have registered patents for immunisation procedures that are claimed to reduce methane emission. They have developed a vaccine containing an antigen derived from rumen methanogenic microorganisms (*Baker, 1998*), and an immunogenic preparation that reduces the activity of rumen protozoa (*Baker et al., 1997*).

Manipulation of the rumen microbial ecosystem : There are many potential opportunities for mitigating methane through microbial intervention in the rumen, such as: targeting methanogens with antibiotics, bacteriocins, or phage; removing protozoa from the rumen; and the development of alternative sinks for hydrogen, such as reductive acetogenesis. All these opportunities are possible through microbial intervention. However, it is very early days in the realisation of these possibilities (*Joblin, 1999*).

Conclusion

1. The best short-term possibility for mitigating methane emissions would seem to be via improvements in animal efficiency.
2. A wide range of feed additives for reducing methane has been tested over the last 40 years. No one has been incorporated into farm practice for many reasons: toxicity, adaptation by the rumen microbes, expense, and lack of a suitable delivery system.
3. Immunisation against methanogens is an interesting concept, but proof of efficacy is not available.

4. Increased understanding of rumen microbiology will be the most likely pathway to control of methanogenesis.
5. Improper management and large number of unproductive and low productive animals are the main cause for methane production in India, thus the breeding strategies can play a significant role in improving the efficiency of Indian livestock to suit the needs.

References

1. Baker S K (1998). Method for Improving Utilisation Nutrients by Ruminants or Ruminant-like Animals. Patent application: international publication number WO 95/11041.
2. Baker S K, Gnanasampanthan G, Purser D B and Hoskinson R M (1997). Immunogenic preparation and method for improving the productivity of ruminant animals. Patent application: international publication number WO 97/00086.
3. Bauman D E, Eppard P J, de Geeter M J and Lanza G M (1985). Responses of high-producing dairy cows to long-term treatment with pituitary somatotrophin and recombinant somatotrophin. Journal of Dairy Science, **68:** 1352-1362.
4. Blaxter K L and Clapperton J L (1965). Prediction of the amount of methane produced by ruminants. British Journal of Nutrition, 19: 511-522.
5. Callaway T R, Martin S A, Wampler J L, Hill N S and Hill G M (1997). Malate content of forage varieties commonly fed to cattle. Journal of Dairy Science, **80:** 1651-1665.
6. Chalupa W (1980). Chemical control of rumen microbial activity. In Digestive Physiology and Metabolism in Ruminants: 325-347. (Eds) Ruckebusch Y & Thivend P. MTP Press, Lancaster, England.
7. Dohme F, Machmuller A, Estermann B L, Pfister P, Wasserfallen A and Kreuzer M (1999). The role of the rumen ciliate protozoa for methane suppression caused by coconut oil. Letters in Applied Microbiology, **29:** 187-192.
8. Gupta R, Chaudhary U B and Chauhan T R (1993). Effect of protein supplementation and defaunation on the growth rate of young buffalo heifers. Indian Journal of Animal Sciences, **63:** 179-183.
9. Joblin K N (1999). Rumen acetogens and their potential to lower ruminant methane emissions. Australian Journal of Agricultural Research, **50:** 1307-1313.

10. Johnson K A and Johnson D E (1995). Methane emissions from cattle. Journal of Animal Science, **73:** 2483-2492.

11. Johnson D E and Johnson K A (2002). Recent Developments in Understanding Enteric Methane Production by Ruminants; Implications for Mitigation. International Non-CO_2 GHG Mitigation Workshop, Washington DC, 2-3 December 2002.

12. Kirchgessner M, Windisch W and Muller H L (1995). Nutritional factors for the quantification of methane production. In Ruminant Physiology: Digestion, Metabolism, Growth and Reproduction: 333-348. (Eds) Engelhardt W, Leonhard-Marek S, Breves G & Gieseke D. Ferdinand Enke Verlag, Stuggart.

13. Krause M (2002). Effect of Malate and Fumarate Supplementation on Methane Production by Ruminal Micro-organisms. Report to AgResearch. 14p.

14. Lassey K R, Ulyatt M J, Martin R J, Walker C F and Shelton I D (1997). Methane emissions measured directly from grazing livestock in New Zealand. Atmospheric Environment, **31:** 2905-2914.

15. Mathison G W, Okine E K, McAllister T A, Dong Y, Galbraith J and Dmytruk O I N (1998). Reducing methane emission from ruminant animals. Journal of Applied Animal Research, **14:** 1-28.

16. Miller T L (1995). Ecology of methane production and hydrogen sinks in the rumen. In Ruminant Physiology: Digestion, Metabolism, Growth and Reproduction: 317-331. (Eds) von Engelhardt W, Leonhard-Marek S, Breves G & Gieseke D. Ferdinand Enke Verlag, Stuttgart.

17. Moss A R, Jouany J P and Newbold J (2000). Methane production by ruminants: its contribution to global warming. Annales de Zootechnie, **49:** 231-253.

18. Van Nevel C J and Demeyer D I (1995). Feed additives and other interventions for decreasing methane emissions. Biotechnology in Animal Feeds and Feeding, **17:** 329-349.

19. Van Nevel C J and Demeyer D I (1996). Control of rumen methanogenesis. Environmental Monitoring and Assessment, **42:** 73-97.

20. Waghorn G C, Tavendale M H and Woodfield D R (2002). Methanogenesis from forages fed to sheep. Proceedings of the New Zealand Grassland Association, **64:** 167-171.

21. Williams D J (1993). Methane emissions from manure of free-range dairy cows. Chemosphere, **26:** 179-187.

22. Woodward S L, Waghorn G C, Ulyatt M J and Lassey K R (2001). Early indications that feeding Lotus will reduce methane emissions from ruminants. In Proceedings of the New Zealand Society of Animal Production, **61:** 23-26.

□□□

6

Methane Mitigation Strategies in Ruminants

Chetna Mahajan*, MPS Tomar and Vikas Mahajan

*Teaching Associate, Department of Veterinary Bio-Chemistry, CVAS, Bikaner

Methane production by ruminants has received global attention due to its contribution to the greenhouse effect and global warming. The global temperature has increased from 0.3 to 0.6^{0}C in the last century and the current trend indicates that it would rise by 1.4-5.8^{0}C and sea level 0.09-0.8mm by the year 2100. The major contributor to the climate change is greenhouse gases (GHG) like methane (CH_4), carbon dioxide ($CO_{2)}$ and nitrous oxide (N_2O). Although most attention has been focussed on CO_2, but CH_4 and N_2O are extremely potent GHGs with methane having 21 fold greater global warming potentials (GWPs) than does CO_2 (Sirohi *et al.*, 2013). Globally, for ruminant systems, N_2O contributes about 49% of the total GWP of emissions and methane about 42%, leaving only 9% contribution of CO_2, therefore reducing CH_4 emissions would have a more rapid effect on the environment.

Livestock is assumed to be responsible for about 80% of total agricultural GHG emissions. Rumen methanogenesis results in the loss of 6-10 per cent of gross energy (GE) intake, or 8-14 per cent of the digestible energy (DE) intake of ruminants (Okine *et al.*, 2004). Mitigation of methane may contribute to lowering the greenhouse effect that is a topical issue for the scientific community (Johnson and Johnson 1995; Moss *et al.*, 2000). Several mechanisms influence the availability of hydrogen in the rumen and subsequent production of enteric methane emissions by ruminants. Therefore, reducing methane (CH_4) production not only improves feed energy use but also enhances the system efficiency.

MECHANISM OF METHANE MITIGATION

There are two mechanisms available by which methane production can be reduced in livestock. These mechanisms influence the availability of H_2 in the rumen and subsequent production of enteric CH_4 emissions by livestock. Processes that yield propionate act as net proton-using reactions. Hence, mitigation strategies aiming at reducing CH_4 production must work towards increasing the propionate production. This will reduce CH_4 production by removing some of the H_2 produced during ruminal fermentation. Another mechanism by which CH_4 production may be reduced during the rumen fermentation process is through the provision of alternative hydrogen acceptors or sinks. In the anaerobic conditions prevailing in the rumen, the oxidation reactions required to obtain energy in the form of ATP release hydrogen. The amount of hydrogen produced is highly dependent on the diet and type of rumen microbes as the microbial fermentation of feeds produces different end products that are not equivalent in terms of hydrogen output.

The H_2 produced in the rumen is critically important to the rumen ecosystem, mainly during the fermentation process. This H_2 removal is extremely important because, if H_2 accumulates, reoxidation of NADH to NAD+ is restricted, and this inhibits carbohydrate degradation, ATP production and microbial growth. Forage digestion and the resultant production of VFA are then restricted (Joblin 1999 and Janssen 2010). In this methanogenesis process, H_2 manipulation in the rumen is the key to controlling methane emissions (Joblin 1999). Strategies need to focus on reducing H_2 production without spoiling digestion, stimulating H_2 use through alternative production pathways for ruminants, and/or archeaea methanogenic inhibition (number and/or activity), associated with stimulation of pathways that consume H_2 to avoid the negative effects of increasing partial H_2 pressure in the rumen.

Strategic reduction of rumen methanogenesis

Methane is commonly referred to as "2H" sink because pairs of protons and electrons are donated and accepted in metabolic reactions. If this process is replaced with an alternative, there is potential to reduce methane emissions and improve energy-use efficiency. Several strategies for utilising hydrogen in the rumen as alternatives to methanogenesis have been identified.

Vegetable oils

Fats and oils change the fermentation process in the rumen, producing more propionic acid and less methane. This enables better digestion of lower quality feed during drier seasons, thereby reducing methane emissions and increasing productivity (Yasothai 2014). Vegetable oils rich in unsaturated fatty acids are saturated in a process called biohydrogenation, carried out mainly by *Butyrivibrio* species (Maia *et al.,* 2007), consuming hydrogen in the process, which makes this process a potential alternate hydrogen sink, since the saturation of a double bond requires 1 mole of hydrogen. The mechanism of action of saturated fatty acids has been related to their ability to damage cell membranes, leading to K+ leakage an indicator of damaged membrane followed by cell death. Furthermore, lipids reduces methane emissions through multiple mechanisms: reduction of fermentable organic matter (lipids are not a source of energy for rumen bacteria); reduction of methanogenic activity due to the presence of medium-chain fatty acids; toxic effects on cellulolytic bacteria (Nagajara *et al.,* 1997) and protozoa (Doreau and Ferlay 1995) due to the effect of polyunsaturated fatty acids (PUFAs) and biohydrogenation of PUFAs. Therefore, effects of specific oil sources on digestibility, rumen fermentation and microbial population need to be assessed.Methane production has been consistently reduced by adding fat or fatty acids to ruminant diets, and it is estimated that fat can reduce methane emissions by 4–5% (g/kg DMI) for every 1 % increase in the fat content of the diet (Grainger and Beauchemin 2011).

The addition of different oils (soya, coconut, canola, rapeseed, etc.) to ruminant diets have been shown to reduce methane production between 19 % and 62 % sheep (Ding *et al.,* 2012), beef cattle (Jordan *et al.,* 2006) and dairy cows (Brask*et al.,* 2013). Narimani-Rad *et al.* (2011) concluded that dietary inclusion of 5% sunflower oil may cause considerable decreases in-vitro gas production parameters and energy indices of mixed ration (40%: forage and 60% concentrated feed) for ruminant. Decreases in gas production potential may be because of prevention of substrate availability for bacteria in SFO included feed or possible toxicity for micro-organism because of SFO fatty acids. Panayakaew *et al.,* 2013 reported coconut and krabok oil supplemented in two doses, providing either 80 (C80 and K80) or 120 mg (C120 and K120) of C12:0 + C14:0 per 100 ml of incubation fluid reduced methane production ($P<0.05$) and increased propionate production ($P<0.05$) at the expense of acetate ($P<0.05$) and butyrate production ($P<0.05$).

Santra *et al.*, 2013 deliberate the effect of four locally available vegetable oils *viz.*, mustard oil, sunflower oil, sesame oil and rice bran oil and found that total rumen protozoa as well as isotrichidae and entodiniomorphid population and methane production decreased ($P<0.01$) due to sunflower oil in the medium. Hidayah *et al.*, 2014 reported the effects of protected vegetable oils (sesame, canola, and flaxseed) supplementation on *in-vitro* fermentation characteristics, rumen microbial population, and methane production in cattle and observed supplementation of calcium soap-flaxseed oil significantly increased total volatile fatty acids (VFA) production, while the supplementation of micro encapsulated flaxseed oil had the highest propionate concentration and H2 utilization, the lowest A:P ratio, and methane production. The effect of supplementary VOs appears to be two-fold, the first acting through inhibition of the activity/viability of the cellulolytic bacteria in therumen, and the second, as a consumer/binder of hydrogen. A study conducted by Mahajan *et al.*, (2016) to assess the effect of carrot seed oil, canola seed oil and rapeseed oil @ 1, 2 and 3% (DM basis) individually on rumen fermentation and methanogenesis *in-vitro* conclusively revealed that the supplementation of diet with rapeseed oil @ 2–3% on dry matter basis had an edge over other oils and levels.Another study conducted by Mahajan *et al.*, (2016) revealed that methane production was the lowest ($P<0.05$) due to cotton seed oil supplementation at 1% level as compared to other vegetable oils (VOs) *viz.*, sunflower seed and castor seed oil on rumen fermentation by using *in-vitro* gas production technique.

Organic acids

Maximizing the flow of metabolic hydrogen (H) in the rumen away from CH_4 and toward volatile fatty acids (VFA) would increase the efficiency of ruminant production and decrease its environmental impact (Ungerfeld *et al.*, 2015). Inclusion of dicarboxylic organic acids in the diet (e.g. malic acid and fumaric acid) results in shifting the rumen fermentation towards propionic acid and hence, lessens methane production (Martin 1998; Lopez *et al.*, 1999a). Itabashi *et al.* (2000) reported that the molar concentration of propionic acid increased with 16% decrease in methane, when Holstein steers were fed with fumaric acid supplemented with salinomycin. However, a 23% reduction in methane emission was reported, when fumaric acid was supplemented along with sorghum silage, whereas, in another study conducted by Newbold *et al.*, 2005, fumarate appeared more effective as a H_2 sink compound. It was calculated to capture 44% of the H_2 previously used for CH_4 formation compared with a 22% capture of H_2 with acrylate. Fumarate also caused stimulation in fibre digestion. Thus, sodium fumarate was recommended as the preferred propionate precursor as a feed ingredient to decrease CH_4 emissions from ruminants. Similarly, Ungerfeld *et al.*, 2007 suggested that fumaric acid at low concentration would be more effective by being converted into propionic acid and hence, reducing methane production.

Li *et al.*, 2009 conducted an *in-vitro* study to investigate the effect of malate or fumarate, when incubated with linolenic acid (á-C18:3) and they concluded that malate and fumarate rechannelled the metabolic H_2 pathway to production of propionate and conjugated linoleic acid CLA, and depressed the process of bio-hydrogenation and methane generation. Linolenic acid alone would also be one of the optimistic alternatives to suppress the CH_4 generation. Li *et al.*, 2010 concluded that malate and fumarate, as propionate precursors, act as alternative electron sinks and can compete with methane generation and bio-hydrogenation of $C_{18:2}$ in the utilization of metabolic hydrogen.5mM fumaric acid addition in diets varying in roughage to concentrate ratio reduced the methane production without affecting dry matter digestibility (Sirohi *et al.*, 2012), whereas, in another similar study, Baraka and Abdul-Rahman (2012) revealed that fumaric acid 0.5 mg/L in combination with two different doses of eugenol, 100, 200 mg were associated with increased propionates at the expense of acetates (low A/P), decreased methane production and increased FE, microbial yield (Y) and VFAs utilization.

Spices and Herbs

Herbs and herbal extracts, such as neem (*Azadirachtaindica*), garlic (*Alliumsativum*), ginger (*Zingiberofficinale*), kadukka (*Terminaliachebula*) and amla (*Emblicaofficinalis*) contain secondary metabolites, such as lignin, tannins, terpenoids, volatile essential oils, alkaloids, etc. have anti-microbial activity and inhibit rumen microbial growth in a very specific way and hence, can be used for selective amelioration of rumen fermentation, especially methanogenesis. Moreover, herbs or their extracts are unlikely to produce any residual effects in the animal products, as they are organic and have been used for centuries by human race without adverse effects (Bunglavan, 2014). In accordance to antimicrobial properties of plant extracts, many studies have focused on their potential for modification of ruminal fermentation during the last decade (Yang *et al.*, 2007; Macheboeuf *et al.*, 2008; Kongmun *et al.*, 2010; Jahani-Azizabadi *et al.*, 2011).The effects of different doses (5, 10 and 20 g/kg) and long-term adaptation of ginger powder on rumen fermentation *in-vivo* in sheep were evaluated by Zhang *et al.*, 2011 and they observed that total volatile fatty acid (VFA) concentration was decreased ($P<0.05$), but the fatty acid compositions, acetate-to-propionate ratio, pH, and ammonia-N concentration were unchanged by the addition of ginger powder. Different plants, herbs and spices (158 samples) were tested in a screening trial to assess their potential to modify ruminal fermentation *in-vitro*, in particular their effectiveness for decreasing methane production. Most of the plants tested did not cause any noticeable effect on the fermentation parameters studied. However, rhizomes and roots of *Rheum officinale* (rhubarb), bark of *Frangulaalnus* (frangula or alder buckthorn) and bulbs of *Alliumsativum* (garlic) decreased methane production and acetate to propionate ratio (Garcia-Gonzalez *et al.*, 2008). Anassori *et al.*, 2011 reported the potential of garlic oil to improve rumen fermentation efficiency through increasing the production of propionate and reducing protozoa population. Hodjatpanah-montazeri *et al.*, 2014 evaluated the effect of 20, 40 and 80 mg/L of cultural fluid of garlic oil (GA20, GA40 and GA80 respectively) and 20, 40 and 80 mg/L of cultural fluid of turmeric extract (TU20, TU40 and TU80 respectively) on rumen fermentation and methane emission and observed a significant reduction in total gas production compared with the control. Furthermore, addition of garlic oil at 80 mg/L strongly decreased methane production during 24 h post incubation (43% lower than the control). Chaudhary and Khan (2012) tested the effects of adding cinnamon, clove, coriander, cumin and turmeric, individually, on the rumen fermentation during their *in-vitro* incubations with wheat for 24 h and observed all spices reduced methane ($P<0.05$) from wheat as compared to the spice-free wheat (control). Coriander reduced methane more followed by turmeric, cumin and cinnamon than the control. Vakilli *et al.*,2013 evaluated the effects of thyme and cinnamon essential oils on feed intake, growth performance, ruminal fermentation and blood metabolites in feedlot calves fed high-concentrate diets and observed decrease in molar proportion of acetate and A:P ratio, whereas the rest of the parameters and blood metabolites showed no change.

Essential Oils

Essential oil has antimicrobial, antibacterial, antifungal and antioxidant properties. Therefore, recently it has been great interest among nutritionist and rumen microbiologist to exploit essential oil as natural feed additives to improve rumen fermentation, inhibition of methanogenesis and efficiency of feed utilization.Addition of plant essential oils, can limit the growth of the micro-organisms participating in methane formation in the rumen, thus resulting in the reduction of its production (Valli *et al.,* 2015). Patra and Yu (2012) evaluated five essential oils (EOs) namely, clove oil (CLO), eucalyptus oil (EUO), garlic oil (GAO), origanum oil (ORO) and peppermint oil (PEO) in-vitro at 3 different doses (0.25, 0.50, and 1.0 g/litre) for their effect on methane production, fermentation, and selected groups of ruminal microbes, including total bacteria, cellulolytic bacteria, archaea and protozoa. All the EOs significantly reduced methane production with increasing doses, with reductions by 34.4%, 17.6%, 42.3%, 87%, and 25.7% for CLO, EUO, GAO, ORO and PEO respectively, at 1.0 g/litre compared with the control. Roy *et al.,* 2014 reported reduction in methane production at 600 ppm dose with supplementation of garlic, oregano, cinnamon and rosemary oils. Sirohi *et al.,*2012 evaluated the efficacy of herbal plant oils Garlic (*Alliumsativum,* GO), Eucalyptus (Eucalyptus globules, EuO) and Neem (*Azadirachtaindica,* NO) on methane reduction. Khiasosa and Zebeli (2013) reported that essential oils and their bioactive compounds at doses <0.75g/kg diet DM acted as a potential methane inhibitor in the rumen as a result of decreased acetate to propionate ratio. Pawar *et al.,* 2014 examined the effect of seven EOs viz. garlic, clove, lemon grass, wild turmeric, turmeric and cinnamon on in-vitro methanogenesis and observed that the lowest level of EOs (167 μl) was the most appropriate level of inclusion for methane inhibition.

Saponins/tannins

Saponins are glycosidic rich compounds decrease methane production in the rumen (Patra and Saxena 2009; Szumzcher-Strabel and Cieslak 2010). The primary effect of saponins in the rumen appears to be to inhibit the protozoa (defaunation), which might increase the efficiency of microbial protein synthesis and protein flow to the duodenum. Furthermore, saponins may decrease methane production via defaunation and/or directly by decreasing the activities (*i.e.,* rate of methanogenesis or expression of methane-producing genes) and numbers of methanogens. Tannins have been found to be toxic for many of the rumen microbes, especially ciliate protozoa, fibre degrading microbes and methanogenic bacteria as a result of this methanogenesis in the rumen is reduced (Valli *et al.*, 2015). Supplementation of phytogenic compounds, such as saponins and tannins were reported to decrease methane emissions in the rumen (Thalib *et al.*, 2004; Jayanegara *et al.*, 2013 and 2014). Sirohi *et al.*, 2014 concluded that saponin fraction of Albizialebbeck has antimethanogenic potential and has an ability to modulate the rumen fermentation parameters. Bharathidhasan *et al.*, 2013 reported that the purified saponin significantly ($P<0.01$) reduced the methane production by 37.6% at 6.2 mg/30ml rumen inoculums than control. However, Yuliana *et al* (2014) revealed that combination of tannin and saponin extracts were potential in mitigating ruminal methane emissions.

Immunization

Methane can also be mitigated by the development of a vaccine that would stimulate the ruminant's immune system to produce antibodies against methane-producing methanogens Wright *et al.*, 2004 developed two vaccines, VF3 (based on three methanogenic strains 1Y, AK-87 and ZA-10) and VF7 (based on seven methanogens), that produced a 7.7 % methane reduction in sheep (g per kg of dry matter intake), despite only approximately 20% of the methanogen population being targeted. They also created a vaccine based on five methanogens (Methanobrevibacter spp. strains 1Y, AK-87, M. millerae ZA-10, Methanomicrobium mobile BP and Methanosphaerastadtmanae MCB-3) that was administered in three vaccinations to sheep (Williams *et al.*, 2009). Surprisingly, immunization with this second vaccine caused methane output to increase by 18%, despite the fact that a larger proportion of the methanogenic population (52%) was targeted. An additional vaccine has recently been developed using subcellular fractions of *Methanobrevibacter ruminantium*M1 (Wedlock *et al.*, 2010). Twenty sheep were vaccinated and then revaccinated three weeks later and the antisera was found to cause agglutination of methanogens and decrease growth and methane production *in-vitro*. The genomic techniques have provided positive clues for probable vaccine targets of methanogens in the rumen (Kumar *et al.*, 2014). Such approaches in future will optimistically lead to methane reducing practices for farm animals.

Conclusion

Efforts are being made by the governments around the world to develop mitigation strategies to reduce CH_4 emissions from ruminant livestock. However, livestock producers are unlikely to adopt these strategies if they reduce animal production and hence, profitability. Therefore, implementation of any strategy must take into account the possible consequences on the efficiency of the entire rumen system. A combination of different methane mitigation strategies should be adopted on farms that show both, nutritional and environmental advantages to the farmers.

References

1. Anassori E, Dalir-Naghadeh B, Pirmohammadi R, Taghizadeh A, Asri-Rezaei S, Maham M, Farahmand-Azar S, Farhoomand P. 2011. Garlic: A potential alternative for monensin as a rumen modifier. *Livestock Science* **142:** 276-287.
2. Baraka T A M and Abdul-Rahman M A. 2012. *In-vitro* evaluation of sheep rumen fermentation pattern after adding different levels of eugenol–fumaric acid combinations. *Veterinary World* **5(2):** 110-117.
3. Bharathidhasan A, Viswanathan K, Balakrishnan V, Valli C, Ramesh S and Senthilkumar S M A. 2013. Effects of purified saponin on rumen methanogenesis and rumen fermentatation characteristics studied using in-vitro gas production technique. *International of Journal Veterinary Science* **2(2):** 44-49.
4. Brask M, Lund P,Weisbjerg M R, Hellwing A L, Poulsen M, Larsen M K and Hvelplund T. 2013. Methane production and digestion of different physical forms of rapeseed as fat supplement in dairy cows. *Journal of Dairy Science* **96:** 2356–2365.
5. Bunglavan S J. 2014. Methanogenesis and recent techniques for mitigation of methanogenesis in ruminants. *Journal of Livestock Science* **5:** 35-48.
6. Chaudhary A S and Khan M M H. 2012. Impacts of different spices on *in-vitro* rumen dry matter disappearance, fermentation and methane of wheat or ryegrass hay based substrates.*Livestock science* **146(1):** 84-90.
7. Ding X, Long R, Zhang Q, Huang X, Guo X and Mi J. 2012. Reducing methane emissions and the methanogen population in the rumen of Tibetan sheep by dietary supplementation with coconut oil. *Tropical Animal Health Production* **44:** 1541–1545.

8. Doreau M and Ferlay A. 1995. Effect of dietary lipids on nitrogen metabolism in the rumen: a review. *Livestock Production Science* **43:** 97-110.

9. Garcia-Gonzalez R, Lopez S, Fernandez M, Bodas R and Gonzale J S. 2008.Screening the activity of plants and spices for decreasing ruminal methane production *in-vitro.Animal Feed Science and Technology* **147:** 36-52.

10. Grainger C and Beauchemin K A. 2011. Can entericmethane emissions from ruminants be lowered without lowering their production? *Animal Feed Science Technology* **166–167:** 308–320.

11. Hidayah N, Suharti S and Wiryawan K G. 2014. In-vitro Rumen Fermentation of Ration Supplemented with Protected Vegetable Oils. *Media Peternakan* **37(2):** 129.

12. Hodjatpanah-montazeri, Mesgaran M D, Vakili A, Ghorbani B and Tabatabaie F. 2014. *In-vitro* Effect of garlic oil and turmeric extract on methane production from gas test medium.*Annual Reviews and Research in Biology* **4(9):** 1439-1447.

13. Itabashi H, Barayu E and Kanda S. 2000. Effect of salinomycin and fumaric acid on rumen fermentation and methane production in cattle. *Asian Australian Journal of Animal Science* **13:** 287.

14. Jahani-Azizabadi H, DaneshMesgaran M, Vakili A, Rezayazdi K, Hashemi M. 2011. Effect of various medicinal plant essential oils obtained from semi-arid climate on rumen fermentation characteristics of a high forage diet using in-vitro batch culture. *African Journal of Microbiology Research* **5(27):** 4812-4819.

15. Janssen P H. 2010. Influence of hydrogen on rumen methane formation and fermentation balances through microbial growth kinetics and fermentation thermodynamics. *Animal Feed Science and Technology* **160:** 1–22.

16. Jayanegara A, Marquardt S, Wina E, Kreuzer M and Leiber F. 2013. *In-vitro* indications for favourable non-additive effects on ruminal methane mitigation between high-phenolic and high-quality forages. *British Journal of Nutrition* **109:** 615-622.

17. Jayanegara A, Wina E and Takahashi J. 2014. Meta analysis on methane mitigating properties of saponin-rich sources in the rumen: influence of addition levels and plant sources. *Asian-Australian Journal of Animal Science* (in press).

18. Joblin K. N. 1999. Rumen acetogens and their potential to lower ruminant methane emissions.*Australian Journal of Agricultural Research* **50(8):** 1307–1313.

19. Johnson K A and Johnson D E. 1995.Methane emissions from cattle.*Journal of Animal Science* **73:** 2483–2492.

20. Jordan E, Kenny D, Hawkins M, Malone R, Lovett D K and O'Mara F P. 2006. Effect of refined soya oil or whole soyabeans on intake, methane output, and performance of young bulls. *Journal of Animal Science* **84(9):** 2418-2425.

21. Khiaosaard R and Zebeli Q. 2013.Meta-analysis of the effects of essential oils and their bioactive compounds on rumen fermentation characteristics and feed efficiency in ruminants. *Journal of Animal Science* **91:** 1819-1830.

22. Kongmun P, Wanapat M, Pakdee P, Nawanukrew C. 2010. Effect of coconut oil and garlic powder on *in-vitro* fermentation using gas production technique. *Livestock Science* **127:** 38–44.

23. Kumar S, Choudhury P K, Carro M D, Griffith G W, Dagar S S, Puniya M, Calabro S, Ravella S R, Dhewa T, Upadhyay R C, Sirohi S K, Kundu S S, Wanapat M K and Puniya A K.2014. New aspects and strategies for methane mitigation from ruminants. *Appl. Microbiol. Biotechnol.,* **98:** 31–44.

24. Li X Z, Long R J, Yan C G, Choi S H, Jin G L and Song M K. 2010. Rumen microbial responses in fermentation characteristics and production of CLA and methane to linoleic acid in associated with malate or fumarate. *Animal Feed Science Technology* **155:** 132–139.

25. Li X Z, Yan C G, Choi S H, Long R J, Jin G L and Song M K. 2009. Effects of addition level and chemical type of propionate precursors in dicarboxylic acid pathway on fermentation characteristics and methane production by rumen microbes *in-vitro*. *Asian-Australian Journal of Animal Science* **22(1):** 82-89.

26. Lopez S, McIntosh F M, Wallace R J and Newbold C J. 1999.Effect of adding acetogenic bacteria on methane production by mixed rumen micro-organisms. *Animal Feed Science Technology* **78:** 1–9.

27. Macheboeuf D, Morgavi D P, Papon Y, Mousset J L, Arturo-Schaan M. 2008. Dose response effects of essential oils on *in-vitro* fermentation activity of the rumen microbial population. *Animal Feed Science Technology* **145:** 335–350.

28. Mahajan C, Mangal K and Wadhwa M. 2016. Effect of addition of vegetable oils on rumen fermentation and methanogenesis under *in-vitro* conditions. *Indian Journal of Animal Nutrition* **33(3):** 296-300.

29. Mahajan C, Mangal K and Wadhwa M. 2016.Effect of vegetable seed oils on methane emission and fermentation of feed *in-vitro. Indian Journal of Animal Sciences* **86(7):** 843–845.

30. Maia M R G, Chaudhary L C, Figueres L and Wallace R J. 2007 Metabolism of polyunsaturated fatty acids and their toxicity to the microflora of the rumen. *Antonie Van Leeuwenhoek* **91:** 303-314.

31. Martin S A. 1998. Manipulation of ruminal fermentation with organic acids: A review. *Journal of Animal Science* **76:** 3123-3132.

32. Moss A R, Jouany J P and Newbold J. 2000. Methane production by ruminants: its contribution to global warming. *Annales dezootechnie.* **49:** 231-253.

33. Nagaraja T G, Newbold C J, Van Nevel C J and Demeyer D I. 1997. Manipulation of ruminal fermentation. *In:* Hobson PN, StewartCS, editors. The rumen microbial ecosystem. London: *Blackie Academic & Professional,* 523-632.

34. Narimani-Rad M, Kiyani N M, Shahryar H A, Maheri-Sis N, Nobar R S and Lotfi A. 2011.Influence of sunflower oil supplementation on in-vitro gas production of mixed ration for ruminants. *European Journal of Experimental Biololgy* **1(4):** 125-129.

35. Newbold C J, Lopez S, Nelson N, Ouda J O, Wallace R J and Moss AR. 2005. Propionate precursors and other metabolic intermediates as possible alternative electron acceptors to methanogenesis in ruminal fermentation *in-vitro. British of Journal of Nutrition* **94:** 27–35.

36. Okine E K, Basarab J A, Laki A, Goonewardene L A, Mir P. 2004. Residual feed intake and feed efficiency: differences and implications. Florida Ruminant Nutrition Symposium. University of Florida. Available at http://dairy.ifas.ufl.edu/files/rns/2004/Okine.pdf [Verified 4 August, 2010]

37. Panyakaew P, Goel G, Lourenc M, Yuangklang C and Fievez V. 2013.Medium-chain fatty acids from coconut or krabok oil inhibit in-vitro Rumen methanogenesis and conversion of non-conjugated dienoicbio hydrogenation. *Animal Feed Science Technology* **180:** 18-25.

38. Patra A K and Yu Z. 2012. Effects of essential oils on methane production and fermentation by, and abundance and diversity of rumen microbial populations. *Applied Environmental Microbiology*

78(12): 4271–4280.

39. Patra K and Saxena J. 2009.The effect and mode of action of saponins on the microbial populations and fermentation in the rumen and ruminant production. *Nutritional Research and Reviews* **22:** 204–219.

40. Pawar M M, Kamra D N, Agarwal N and Chaudhary L C. 2014. Effects of essentials oils on *in-vitro* methanogenesis and feed fermentation with buffalo rumen liquor. *Agriculture Research* **3(1):** 67-74.

41. Santra A, Banerjee and Das S K. 2013.Effect of vegetable oils on ciliate protozoa, methane yield, enzyme profile and rumen fermentation *in-vitro. Animal Feed Science Technology* **13:** 181-193.

42. Sirohi S K, Chaudhary P P, Singh N, Singh D and Puniya A K. 2013. The 16SrRNA and mcrA gene based comparative diversity of methane genes in cattle fed on high fibre based diet. *Gene* **523:** 161-166.

43. Sirohi S K, Goel N and Singh N. 2014. Influence of albizia lebbeck saponin and its fractions on *in-vitro* gas production kinetics, rumen methanogenesis, and rumen fermentation characteristics. *ISRN Veterinary Science* 1-9.

44. Sirohi S K, Mehta M, Goel N and Pandey P. *2012.* Effect of herbal plants oil addition in total mixed diets on anti-methanogenic activity, rumen fermentation and gas production kinetics *in-vitro. Journal of Natural Products and Plant Resources* **2(1):** 73-80.

45. Szumacher-Strabel M and Cieslak A. 2010.Potential of phytofactors to mitigate rumen ammonia and methane production. *Journal of Animal Feed Science* **9:** 319–337.

46. Thalib A. 2004. *In-vitro* study of effectiveness of saponin from *Sapindus rarak* fruit as methanogenesis inhibitor on ruminal digestion system. JITV **9:** 164-171.

47. Ungerfeld E M, Kohn R A, Wallace R J, Newbold C J. 2007. A meta-analysis of fumarate effects on methane production in ruminal batch cultures. *Journal of Animal Science* **85:** 2556–2563.

48. Ungerfeld E M. 2015. Shifts in metabolic hydrogen sinks in the methanogenesis-inhibited ruminal fermentation: a meta-analysis. *Frontiers in microbiology* **6:** 1.

49. Vakili A R, Khorrami B, Danesh Mesgaran, M and Parand, E. 2013. The effects of thyme and cinnamon essential oils on performance, rumen fermentation and blood metabolites in Holstein Calves Consuming High Concentrate Diet. *Asain Australas. J. Anim. Sci.* **26(7):**

935-944.

50. Valli C, Bungalavan M, Ramachandran S J and Balakrishnan V. 2015. Methane emission from ruminants and utility of plant extracts in reduction of methanogenesis. *Indian Journal of Veterinary Animal Science Research* **44(1):** 78-88.

51. Wedlock D N, Pedersen G, Denis M, Dey D, Janssen P H and Buddle B. M. 2010. Development of a vaccine to mitigate green house gas emissions in agriculture: vaccination of sheep with methanogen fractions induces antibodies that block methane production *in-vitro*. *New Zealand Veterinary Journal* **58(1):** 29–36.

52. Williams Y J, Popovski S, Rea S M, Skillman L C, Toovey A F, Northwood K S, Wright A D. 2009. A vaccine against rumen methanogens can alter the composition of archaeal populations. *Applied Environmental Microbiology*, **75:** 1860–1866.

53. Wright A D G, Kennedy P, O'Neill C J. Toovey A, Popovski S, Rea S, Pimm C and Klein L 2004. Reducing methane emissions in sheep by immunization against rumen methanogens. *Vaccine* **22:** 3976–3985.

54. Yang W Z, Benchaar C, Ametaj B N, Chaves A V, He M L, McAllister T A. 2007. Effects of garlic and juniper berry essential oils on ruminal fermentation and on the site and extent of digestion in lactating cows. *Journal of Dairy Science* **90:** 5671–5681.

55. Yasothai R. 2014.Reducing methanogenesis in ruminants. *Universal Journal of Pharmacy* **3(05):** 32-35.

56. Yuliana P, Laconi1 E B, Wina E and Jayanegara A. 2014. Extraction of tannins and saponins from plant sources and their effects on *in-vitro* methanogenesis and rumen fermentation. *Journal of Indonesian tropical Animal Agriculture* **39(2):** 91-97.

57. Zhang T T, Yang Z B, Yang W R, Jiang S Z and Zhang G G. 2011. Effects of dose & adaptation time of ginger root (Zingiberofficinale) on fermentation. *Journal of Animal Feed Science* **20:** 461–471.

□□□

7

Livestock, Externalities and the Environment

Vijay Kumar Sharma*, Amrish Vaid, Pawan Kumar Sharma, Brijesh Ajrawat, Anamika Jamwal, Vishal Mahajan and Saurav Gupta

* KVK, Kathua, SKUAST-Jammu

India is often criticized for the negative externalities to the ecology due to the largest livestock population of the country. Thus, inspite of the fact that the integrated farming system followed in the country contributes towards not only saving the resources and improving the environment. This study quantifies the positive environmental externalities associated with the livestock production in the context of integrated farming system of rainfed areas. It included land saving due to recycling of agricultural by-products as animal feed and also due to use of dung- cake as domestic fuel, saving of chemical fertilizers due to use of dung as manure and prevention of carbon dioxide emission due to use of animal energy in agriculture.

India being one of the largest livestock keeper of the world, its livestock sector comes under the stringent scrutiny of the global climate monitoring agencies, such as IPCC. This inspite their significant contributions towards enhancing food and nutritional security are often criticized for the negative externalities they cause to environment through emission of green house gases, overgrazing/ deforestation and water pollution. According to the estimates of the Indian Network for Climate Change Assessment, the agricultural sector emitted 334 Mt of CO_2 in 2007, to which livestock contributed about 63 per cent. Further, livestock contribute 18 per cent of global green house gas (GHG) emissions (Steinfeld *et al.*, 2006). Apart from enteric emission decomposition of livestock manure under anaerobic conditions is also a source of methane. Another green house gas is nitrous oxide (N_2O), released during the nitrification-denitrification of nitrogen contained in livestock waste. Cattle and feedlots are responsible for 26% of N_2O emissions from anthropogenic sources (IPCC, 2001). Being green house gases their large scale emission is detrimental to the environmental safety. So, different strategies are emerging to either subside their emission from faeces and animal wastes or to use them effectively for energy saving purposes. A number of studies in the past have quantified methane emission from livestock production. These studies have shown wide variations, ranging from 8.5 Mt to 10.5 Mt, depending on the methods and data used and also the year for which the gas emission was estimated (Lerner *et al.*, 1988; Ahuja, 1990; Bhattacharya and Mitra, 1998; Mishra and Dikshit, 2004; Singhal *et al.*, 2005; Swamy and Bhattacharya, 2006; Singh *et al.*, 2012). Negative externalities of livestock to environment are well documented and quantified (Steinfeld *et al.*, 2006) but their positive contributions have remained less documented and non-quantified. The prominent positive environmental contributions include prevention of carbon dioxide emission due to use of animal energy in place of fossil fuel, saving of natural resources mainly land as a result of recycling of agricultural by-products and residues as animal feed, and dung in place of firewood as domestic fuel and as a substitute for chemical fertilizers.

Estimation of Feed Consumption Rates

Household level feed consumption rates serve as a base to estimate feed consumption rates at the national level. From the survey, we gathered information on (i) number of sample households having livestock, say cattle in milk and (ii) number of cattle in-milk observed, and (iii) amount of feed fed per day to these cattle in-milk. We then scaled-up information.

Utilisation of land saving because of recycling of crop residues as animal feed

1By using the feed consumption rates, we can quantify the positive contributions of livestock production systems to the environment following the "Environmental Model of Livestock Production System" by Mishra and Dikshit (2004).

The estimated positive impact of the system included land saving due to crop by-product used as animal feed, and due to use of dung as a domestic fuel; saving in chemical fertilizers due to dung-use as a manure; saving in fossil fuel (diesel) due to use of animal energy in agricultural operations. The model has been described as follows:

The gross energy intake per animal per day from by-product feed was estimated by summing up the energy values of by-product feed on dry matter basis. Similarly, the energy value of green fodder fed to the animals was also calculated on dry matter basis. Then, the annual quantity of green fodder required, in terms of energy to replace gross energy from by-product feed, was estimated as per equation (1) :

$$G_f = \left[\frac{1}{e} \times gei \times \frac{1}{d} \right] \times 365$$

where, Gf is the quantity of green fodder required to replace the by-product feed, gei is the gross energy intake from by-product feed (dry fodder and concentrates), e stands for the energy (million calories) per unit of Gf; and d is the dry matter fraction of green fodder. We then estimated the land area required to produce Gf. Let y be the yield of green fodder per hectare of land, then the area L required to produce Gf may be given by equation (2):

$$L = \frac{G_f}{y} \quad \text{...(2)}$$

Land Saving due to Use of Dung as Substitute for Firewood in Domestic Fuel

In rural households, firewood is used as a domestic fuel; for cultivation or perennial firewood trees cover land and deprive its use for farming. The use of dung cake as firewood would result in the saving of this land, which can be used for crop-cultivation. We, therefore, estimated the land saved due to use of dung cake as a domestic fuel. The dung-cake output on dry matter basis was worked out using dung evacuation rate and its dry matter fraction. Supposing o as the rate of substitution of dry fuel-wood for dung cake (fuel-wood: dry dung cake) in terms of thermal energy, the total quantity of dry fuel-wood required to replace the supply (output) of dung cake was calculated by equation (3):

$$Fw = \delta \times dc \quad \text{...(3)}$$

where, Fw is the quantity of fuel-wood required to replace dung cake, and dc is the quantity of dung cake output. Now, let us suppose that fuel-wood is produced and used within the year, and its yield per hectare on dry matter basis is y, then the total land area that would be required for producing Fw can be calculated by equation (4):

$$L = \frac{1}{y} \times Fw \qquad \ldots(4)$$

The effect of gestation lag in the production of fuel wood can be described as follows:

The model assumes that fuel-wood is produced and used within the same year. This is apparently an unrealistic assumption. In reality, more than one year is required to cover the whole process of fuel-wood tree plantation, growth and logging of trees, drying and use of cut-out wood as fuel. Suppose it takes 3 years to complete the process before dry wood is made available for use at the end of the 3rd or the beginning of 4th year. This means that, whereas the fuel wood made available can replace equivalent amount of dung cake only in the fourth year, the necessary land area required for growing and harvesting of trees for making the fuel-wood available will have to be kept locked up during the preceding 3 years. This implies that around 3-times as much land will be required or saved if one year's dung cake output was used in place of fuel wood as energy source.

Saving of Chemical Fertilizers due to Use of Dung as Manure

The extent to which dung manure substitutes the chemical fertilizers, is a saving of chemical fertilizers. Fresh cattle dung on an average contains 0.30-0.40 per cent nitrogen (N), 0.10-0.20 per cent phosphorus (P_2O_5), and 0.10-0.30 per cent potassium oxide (K_2O) (Anonymous, 1997). According to the recent estimates of Ghosh *et al.* (2004), dung manure contains 0.71 per cent N, 0.18 per cent P_2O5 and 0.71 per cent K_2O. In this study, we have used the fraction of soil nutrients (N,P and K) in dung-manure as estimated by Ghosh *et al.* (2004), and the total quantity of N, P and K was worked out for the proportion of bovine dung used as manure.

Saving of Fossil Fuel due to Animal Energy-use in Agriculture

If the working animals were to be replaced by agricultural machinery, it would require additional fuel and lead to emission of CO_2 from burning of the fossil fuel. It is this emission that is prevented by the livestock. It has been assumed in the study that tractors are the only machine used and are of similar power; and also the working animals do not differ in their work capacity. In order to determine the saving of fossil fuel and prevention of green house gasses due to animal energy use, we need to know (i) the rate of substitution between tractors and working animals, (ii) the amount of diesel required for running a tractor to perform agricultural operations, and (iii) the amount of CO_2 that will be emitted from the burning of a unit of diesel. On the basis of economic substitution rate, 10 working males are required to replace a tractor. The number of tractors required for replacing country's bovine working stock, diesel use, and the associated emission of green house gases have been estimated.

From time to time not only international organisations but also developed countries target India for its large livestock population. Thus, a number of the studies were undertaken to quantify the methane emission from Indian livestock. These studies showed large variations ranging from 8.5 Mt to 10.5 Mt, depending upon the methods used as well as the period of the study (Lerner *et al.*, 1988; Ahuja, 1990; Bhattacharya and Mitra, 1998; Mishra and Dikshit, 2004; Singhal *et al.*, 2005; Swamy and Bhattacharya, 2006; Singh *et al.*, 2012). Inspite of the various negative externalities attributed, integrated farming system of the rainfed system contributes towards the contributes towards reducing the chemical fertilizers and carbon dioxide emissions.

Conclusion

Extension interventions have importance to reduce negative externalities of livestock besides popularising technologies for increasing productivity and further popularising animal diets that would result reduction in methane emissions.

References

1. Ahuja, D. (1990). United State Environmental Agency (USEPA), *Inventory of U.S. Green house Gas Emissions and Sink*, 1990-98.

2. Anonymous (1997). *Hand Book of Agriculture,* Indian Council of Agriculture Research (ICAR), New Delhi.
3. Bhattacharya, S. and Mitra, A.P. (1998). *Green house Gas Emission in India for the Base Year 1990.* Scientific Report, No.11, Centre for Global Change, National Physical Laboratory, New Delhi.
4. Ghosh, P.K. et al. (2004) Comparative effectiveness of cattle manure, poultry manure, phosphor compost and fertilizer-NPK on three cropping systems in Vertisols of semi-arid tropics, *Crop Yields and System Performance,* **95:** 77-83.
5. IPCC (Inter-Governmental Panel on Climate Change) (1995) *Revised IPCC Guidelines for National Green house Gas Inventories,* OECD, Paris.
6. Lerner, J., Mathews, E. and Fung, I. (1988) Methane emission from animals, a global high resolution data, *Global Biogeochemical Cycles,* **2**: 139-156.
7. Mishra, S.N. and Dikshit, A.K. (2004) *Environment and Livestock in India : With a Comparative Study of the Indian and US Dairy Systems,* Manohar Publishers and Distributors, New Delhi.
8. Singh, S., Kushwaha, B.P., Nag, S.K., Bhattacharya, S., Gupta, P.K., Mishra, A.K. and Singh, A. (2012) Assessment of enteric methane emission of Indian livestock in different agro-ecological regions, *Current Science,* **102(7):** 1017-1027.
9. Singhal, K.K., Mohini, M., Jha, A. K. and Gupta, P.K. (2005) Methane emission estimates from enteric fermentation in Indian livestock: Dry matter intake approach, *Current Science,* **88:** 119-127.
10. Steinfeld, H., Gerber, P., Wassennar, T., Castel, V., Rosales, M. and de Haan, C. (2006) *Livestock's Long Shadow: Environmental Issues and Options,* Food and Agriculture Organization of the United Nations, Rome.
11. Swamy, M. and Bhattacharya, S. (2006) Budgeting anthropogenic green house gas emission from Indian livestock using country-specific emission coefficients, *Current Science,* **91:** 1340-1353.

□□□

8

Management Strategies for Conservation of Indigenous Poultry by Molecular Approach

Prabhat Kumar Pankaj*, R.K. Mahapatra, R. Pourouchottamane and Vikas Mahajan

* ICAR-Central Research Institute for Dryland Agriculture, Santoshnagar, Hyderabad-500059 (Telangana State)

Poultry plays an important role in rural livelihood security as well as is an integral part of human life in many ways by providing animal protein as meat and eggs. In drylands, especially Andhra Pradesh and Tamilnadu, they has social and ethical value through hobby, sporting, etc. There is an excellent advancement in poultry production through extensive usage of population genetics principles and intensive selection and development of specialized populations of poultry. For continued genetic progress, it is very important to conserve the genetic reservoir of existing poultry populations which can respond to future research and production needs in a sustainable way. Like other species, poultry biodiversity is also declining at an alarming level globally and we may need to review the urgency of conserving poultry biodiversity because avian species are unique and the topic becomes more important in the era of climate change.

Nearly 36% of meat production in India is contributed by poultry and 12.82% of total egg production is from Desi Fowls (BAHS, 2016). The largest producer of egg is Tamilnadu which produces 19.4% of the total egg production in the country followed by Andhra Pradesh that produces 18.89% of the egg production. Telangana is the third largest egg producer state in the country which produces 13.5% of the total egg production in the country (BAHS, 2016).

Poultry is reared by marginal and small farmers due to its low feed, water and other production input requirements and thus, contributes significantly to the rural livelihoods and economy.

However, indigenous breeds are very important in the period of climate change where temperature, humidity, rainfall and climatic extreme events are uncertain and more frequent. Indigenous breeds of India are more hardy, agile to escape from predators, adapted to varied agro-ecosystem, greater capacity to be reared on low grade feed materials, hard egg shell and having good nutritive valued meat. To achieve the fast growth in poultry sector with higher FCR, better genomic research in this area is need of the hour. To meet the growing demands of the population and to improve the per capita consumption among the rural/tribal people, indigenous poultry farming in rural/tribal areas is the best alternative. Indigenous chickens are of great importance to smallholder farmers in India and it requires the challenge towards improving productivity for increasing financial and food security.

Thus, current concept deals with management strategies for conservation of indigenous poultry by molecular approach in detail.

Poultry Genetic Resources in India, its Diversification and Conservation Needs

The breeds of poultry in India are locally adapted and evolved over years altogether, but have been replaced indiscriminately by crossbred or pure stocks at a faster rate due to its increasing demand, industrialization and development in secondary agriculture. Their productivity, phenotypic characteristics, food value and true genetic potentials are lesser known areas. The small poultry holders are non-competitive now due to economic reasons. India has 28 recognized poultry breeds of India (http://www.nbagr.res.in/regchi.html). These indigenous birds are primarily reared as backyard poultry and have their utility in egg, meat and game. These indigenous birds are poor layers producing 40-60 eggs per year. Apart from them, there are other non-descript indigenous poultry breeds which also need attention and conservation.

An assessment of genetic diversity using molecular markers may serve as a initial guide to identify unique and valuable genetic resources as geographical isolation has never been followed in India. Such attempts have been made using several molecular tools (Oka *et al.*, 2007; Muchadeyi *et al.*, 2008 and Silva *et al.*, 2009) using microsatellite technique (autosomal markers) and mt DNA (maternally inherited), single nucleotide polymorphisms (SNPs) assessment for insights into diversity within and between indigenous poultry populations. Such studies will indicate the variability in the population and will suggest about the conservation requirements. Also, maintaining local genetic resources are needed to permit genetic adaptation of populations to unforeseen breeding requirements in the future and as a source of research material (Besbes, 2009).

For conserving the diversity, two tools of conservation (prevention of breed extinction and management of genetic diversity) is used. Local breed conservation has two-fold benefit of ensuring livelihoods of farmers who rear them and they could become future assets in breeding programs. Means to preserve the important and unique characteristics of Indian local poultry genetic resources should be encouraged.

Molecular Techniques Helpful in Conservation of Breeds

Major genes of breeding importance in poultry of India with special utility are blue shell (O), dwarf (Dw), fibro-melanosis (Fm), frizzle (E), naked neck (Na), non-inhibitor (Id), pea comb (P), silky (H) and slow feathering (K). A wide diversity of indigenous poultry breeds in India could form the basis for genetic improvement and diversification adapted to specific environments and requirements.

Major advantages of using highly polymorphic markers are their locus specificity, abundance and random distribution over the genome, co-dominant inheritance, ease and speed of their application and suitability for semi-automated analysis (Weigend and Romanov, 2001). Genetic diversity within a breed can be estimated by the number of alleles, the expected heterozygosity (Frankham *et al.*, 2002) and marker estimated kinships within a breed (Eding and Meuwissen, 2001). Genetic diversity between breeds can be assessed using genetic distances (Reynolds *et al.*, 1983). However, a holistic approach to assess genetic diversity within and between populations can be made on the basis of marker estimated kinships (Eding and Meuwissen, 2001) or Bayesian clustering approaches (Pritchard *et al.*, 2000).

In an analysis of the poultry population structure, Granevitze *et al.* (2007) found six main clusters which were related to their geographical origins and histories. These six main clusters were formed by 1) brown egg layers, 2) predominantly broilers, 3) native Chinese breeds or breeds with recent Asian origin, 4) predominantly breeds of European derivation, 5) populations with no known history, and 6) the other populations shared their genome with some clusters defined as "Multi-clusters". The various molecular techniques used in conservation tools are as follows:

1. Molecular markers

Used for determining the genetic variation and biodiversity with high levels of accuracy and reproducibility. They are classified into two types: mitochondrial and nuclear markers. The most commonly used nuclear markers for DNA fingerprinting include random amplified polymorphic DNA (RAPD), amplified fragment length polymorphism (AFLP) and microsatellites. The important characteristics of mtDNA are maternal lineage, degradation slower than nuclear DNA, used in degraded samples and evolves about 10–fold faster than nuclear DNA; 12s rDNA is highly conserved and used for high category phyla and subphyla; 16S rDNA is used in mid-category differentiation; Control region is hypervariate and used for identification of species and sub-species; Protein-coding genes are conserved and used in low-categories.

1.1. Nuclear DNA markers

a) *Microsatellites :* are multiple copies of short tandem repeats (1–5 base pair (bp) long), located in both, coding and non-coding regions and fairly evenly distributed throughout the eukaryotic genomes. They are highly polymorphic, abundant and can easily be amplified by polymerase chain reaction (PCR), rendering them highly versatile markers for molecular fingerprinting.

b) *SNPs :* have rather low information content, and larger numbers have to be used to reach the level of information obtained from a standard panel of 30 microsatellite loci, however, increasing automation may reduce the cost. SNPs can be generated through various experimental protocols, such as sequencing, single-stranded conformational polymorphism (SSCP) or denaturing high-performance liquid chromatography (DHPLC), or *in silico*, aligning and comparing multiple sequences of the same region from public genome and expressed sequence (EST) databases.

c) *AFLPs :* Are dominant biallelic markers and are highly informative in assessing the relationship between breeds and related species.

1.2. Mitochondrial DNA markers (mtDNA)

They have been extensively used in phylogenetic and genetic diversity analyses as well as for species level identification using DNA barcoding. The polymorphisms in the sequence of the hypervariable region of the D-loop or control region of mtDNA have contributed greatly to the identification of the wild progenitors of domestic species, the establishment of geographic patterns of genetic diversity, and the understanding of livestock domestication (Bruford *et al.*, 2003).

2. DNA barcoding

Is used to identify and distinguish biological species based on its unique identity carried in its DNA molecules. DNA sequence analysis of a uniform target gene to enable species identification has been termed DNA barcoding. The Consortium for the Barcode of Life (*http://barcoding.si.edu*) is a worldwide initiative devoted to develop an accurate and reliable tool for scientific research on the identification of plant and animal species.

3. D-loop (Control region) of mt genome

The mtDNA control region is the only large non-coding region in avian mitochondria which contains heavy-strand replication origin and the promoters for both the L- and H-strand transcription. The central domain is the most conserved and contains several structural elements (B, C-, D- and E- boxes) that can be readily aligned even between different bird families.

The control region is highly variable in birds and thus, evolves faster than the rest of the mt genome which makes it useful for population structure to phylogenetic relationship studies. This region is helpful in elucidating the global population structure in poultry. Thus, D-loop of mtDNA has wide application in poultry genetics including the study of genetic diversity, population structure, evolutionary relationships and identification of species with exploration of global migration. Hyper variability of primary structure in the control region of mitochondrial DNA (mtDNA) in different poultry populations can serve the basis for their effective identification and designing of stock structure. A low genetic variation in D-loop sequences among the individuals of a species potentially indicates that the organism had undergone a severe bottleneck in the past.

Conservation of Indigenous Poultry Genetic Resources

Poultry genetic resources are considered to be the most endangered with the highest proportion of breeds (33%) at risk. The main factors responsible for depletion of indigenous poultry genetic resources are low performance of local breeds, farmers' preferences for exotic breeds, the lack of adequate conservation policies, socio-economic changes, natural and human induced disasters, and the transformation of traditional systems into external input-oriented systems (FAO, 2007).

One of the important objectives of conservation programs is to maintain genetic diversity for potential future use. Eding and Bennewitz (2007) indicated two different methods using molecular genetic variation to derive conservation priorities which are the core set (Eding *et al.*, 2002) and a widely used formal approach for decision making in livestock conservation based on Weitzman's (1992) diversity concept. Conservation potential is considered as the single most useful breed alert indicator in conservation decision (Weitzman, 1993). Conservation potentials were applied for prioritizing poultry (Pinent *et al.*, 2005) breeds. The populations in these studies showed a considerable variability of their conservation potentials. Although migration between breeds or within breed diversity is neglected applying the Weitzman approach as criticized by Caballero and Toro (2002) and Eding et al. (2002), decisions on investments in conservation based on the Weitzman approach are driven not only by the phylogenetic substructure, but also by economic and social factors, which serve as an important consideration in the conservation decisions (FAO, 2007). Weitzman diversity for conservation can maintain allelic diversity within species, ensuring maximum adaptive potential of species (Simianer, 2005 and Tapio *et al.*, 2006) since conservation activities aim to reduce the extinction probability and to increase expected diversity of populations as suggested by Simianer (2005) and FAO (2007). Conservation strategies needs to understand how the available resources should be dispersed among the breeds and its efficiency (FAO, 2007). In most cases, national conservation programs financially support farmers to maintain their breeds despite the economic inferiority of their breeds. Such a low allocation might not ensure to prevent the loss of national animal germplasm resources in the long term (Tieu *et al.*, 2008).

Breeding strategies

To efficiently exploit the potential of indigenous local germplasm and to be sustainable, long term vision with flexible approach and responsive to variable factors. Designing a breeding programme is more than just increased productivity. It should be integrated with infrastructure, community development, improved livelihood and biodiversity, agricultural development policy, environment, production system and market. Similarly, required integration of all activities, adequate training of the personnel and incentives to run the breeding programme successfully is often ignored. There is no better way of conserving a breed for future use than keeping it viable commercially or culturally through a demand-driven and efficient long term breeding programme.

Changing the breeding animal for every 2-3 years (male animal exchange from other district herd) or artificial insemination with proven breed semen will not only help in enhancing the productivity (Pankaj *et al.,* 2013) but also maintain the heterogeneity. This may be supplemented with supply of superior males through formation of nucleus herd at village level. Synchronization of breeding period depending on the availability of feed and fodder resources results in healthy offsprings and better weight gain. Concentrate mixture supplementation to breeding animals should be initiated at least 1 month before breeding season and continued till the weaning. Local climate resilient breeds of moderate productivity should be promoted over susceptible crossbreds.

In developing countries with small herd sizes, large fluctuations in rearing conditions and management between herds, and over time within a herd, lack of systematic livestock identification, inadequate recording of livestock performances and pedigrees, and constraints related to the subsistence nature of livestock rearing (where monetary profit is not the most important consideration), the accuracy of selection will be much lower resulting in even lower rates of genetic gain. However, locally adapted breeds are likely to be highly variable and the highest performing animals of such breeds shall have great productive potential. Therefore, the screening of livestock populations previously not subjected to systematic selection is likely to give quicker results to provide high genetic merit foundation stock for nucleus flocks.

Cross-breeding with a more productive breed can yield faster improvement. However, an appropriate improver breed has to be available, which will adapt to the conditions, where it is to be introduced. If it is a completely new introduction, it is better to conduct a trial and monitor the performance of crosses for a few years before undertaking large-scale crossbreeding programme. There are many other considerations, such as ensuring supply of good quality animals of the improver breed, livestock keepers' acceptance of the improver germplasm, a distribution strategy of breeding males or semen, and a strategy for maintenance of the local breed so that it is not displaced completely by the crosses. Financial consideration is also important because it could be expensive to import the improver breed.

Improvements in components of livestock production other than genetics are more effective and successful in improving incomes and livelihoods if they are accompanied by genetic upgradation. One important consideration for breeding in the changed climate is to whether match the genotypes with the environment or the other way round. There are two main approaches: one is modifying the environment making it less harsh, and the other is to select stock which is most adaptable to the prevailing conditions. In most of traditional livestock production system of developing countries, it has been experienced that existing level of management, nutrition and veterinary care are not sufficient to support the production potential of improved breeds. Further, the extent to which the variables like climate, disease, pasture and associated nutrition, are modifiable will determine the approach. Cost-benefit analysis and application of both the avenues as per requirement shall be the norm. For this purpose, thorough understanding of genetic constitution of the animal population and how it interacts with environment is required. Since not many determinant of environment can be changed in a low-input tropical production system, identification of production system and the finding the best match for it, will be the best choice. Prima-facie, utilization of best locally available and adapted genotypes with improvements in environment to the extent feasible and economical, is going to be the choice. For this the most productive and adapted animals for each environment need to be identified for breeding purposes.

It is debatable whether to select animals for important traits, e.g. production, reproduction along with adaptive traits in harsh environment. It is evident that physiological adaptability is expressed on performance, hence the question arises whether selection of animal on the basis of performance in given environment (stressors) alone will be sufficient or not. Favourable correlation suggests that if we place major importance on performance traits (e.g. reproduction, growth, etc.) in stressful environments, adaptability traits would not be compromised and will lead selection of most favourable animals. Addition of adaptive traits as such might not be of that rewarding because firstly, estimates of heritability of adaptability traits in most of the population is not available; secondly, since genetic correlation between adaptive and productive traits are normally not very high, genetic progress for individual traits may slow down with inclusion of additional traits.

Regarding designing a sustainable breeding programme, it must be set in relation to the resources available and the stage of development the action area concerned. It also needs to be integrated with farmer participation. The design may vary depending on breed, production system or other circumstances.

The breeding objective at micro-level will be determined by relative importance assigned to different traits in the given production environment while macro-level will be determined by agricultural development policy, market, production system and output required from the system in the locality, region or the country, for the longer time horizon. While the long-term goals determine the breeding objectives and relative importance of each trait, the short-term benefits for farmers must be considered to confirm farmer participation. It might be difficult to exactly value the change in all desired traits in economic terms; fundamental traits must always be considered in the selection programme, e.g., through independent culling or other appropriate methods if the indexing method does not work. Special care must be taken to give due importance to fitness and adaptive traits.

The choice of breeding method, i.e. pure breeding or crossbreeding, is the most important decision to be undertaken during the designing the breeding programme. The important factors that will determine it are performance level and potential of genetic improvement in indigenous breeds through selection, availability of alternate breeds for crossbreeding along with their performance and adaptability, heterosis for the major traits, the availability and feasible expansion of infrastructures to maintain two or more pure breeds for long-term crossbreeding programme, cost-benefit analysis of crossbreeding over within breed selection or whether a synthetic breed will be better alternate to pure bred or crossbred.

Conservation strategies

Conservation of biodiversity among poultry genetic resources will bring species specific understanding within their boundaries, especially those which are rare or endangered, or that are characteristic of the region, ecosystem, or location. Active consideration for management of conservation biodiversity in changing climatic scenario will help to regain the gene pool of animal genetic resource.

In–situ conservation strategies

Conservation of animal genetic resources in local climate or the climate as near to its native breeding tract is referred as *In-situ* conservation. The strategy for In-situ conservation includes:

- Proper survey and monitoring of animal genetic resource in the native tract of animals
- Development of organized herd/farm in farmers' field
- Formation of breeders' society
- Development of organized breeding farm by government organization
- Implementation of herd registration scheme

Ex–situ conservation strategies

This is the conservation strategy for maintaining the animal gene pool away from its breeding tract. *Ex-situ* conservation strategies should be developed for the endangered or near-to-extinct group of animals by following two methods:

In-vivo conservation strategy refers to maintaining fewer numbers of live animals away from its breeding tract like different breed specific farm of zoological garden. However, this is mostly followed in case of wild animal conservation.

In-vitro conservation is a type of ex-situ conservation strategy, wherein the genetic material of animals is kept in form of frozen condition for longer duration of time. Long time preservation of gene pool in form of frozen semen and cryopreserved oocyte or embryo is the major strategies of *in-vitro* conservation. Development of DNA data bank, c-DNA library of different animal genetic resources will also help to conserve the vital gene pool.

Production management strategies

The means to maintain the biodiversity and conservation of breed through production management strategies are as follows:

- Agro-forestry systems have substantial potential to sequester carbon and can reduce soil erosion, moderate climate extremes on crops, improve water quality, and provide alternate income and fuel to local people. Agro-forestry can greatly increase biodiversity, especially in landscapes dominated by annual crops or on lands that have been degraded. The plantings can be used to functionally link forest fragments and other critical habitat as part of a broad landscape management strategy.
- Farmers have evolved the farming systems and the strategies that are compatible with the specific resource features of the ecosystems over millennia. Common property resources (CPRs), mainly the community lands under forests and grasslands, have been central to these strategies. Their access to and control over CPRs, which are often exceptionally rich in natural biodiversity, makes them resource-rich and ensures survival and sustainability of their systems and life. Ecological niches full of exceptionally high-value biodiversity including that in the CPRs, and genetic resources in the farmlands, would be the basis for the sustainability of ecosystems.
- The biophysical resource base - land, soil, water sources, forest ecosystems, and agro-biodiversity, is basic to the sustainability of food production and livelihoods in the rural areas. Forest-cropland ratio must be as wide enough as possible (dense forest area, in order to provide a sound ecological balance and natural subsidy to farmland, must be at least five times larger than the cropland area) (Singh, 2004).
- Flow of water and moisture circulation within a farming system is vital for the sustenance of all forms of life. Availability of water in the system also ensures higher level of food production.
- Farmers rear all types of animals, that are suitable for the farming systems. They achieve functional diversity through combining complementary plant and animal species in synergetic interactions, injecting sustainability into the agro-ecosystems. By transferring nutrients from forest ecosystem to farmlands and maintaining cyclic flow pattern in the farming system, they

contribute to the ecological integrity of the system. High degree of biodiversity creates barriers against any natural calamity and pest epidemics.

- Some miscellaneous activities that promote mitigation of or adaptation to climate change as well as help in support system of conservation of breeds include:
  - Maintaining and restoring native ecosystems,
  - Protecting and enhancing ecosystem services,
  - Managing habitats for endangered breeds/species,
  - Creating refuges and buffer zones, and
  - Establishing networks of terrestrial, freshwater and marine protected areas that take into account projected changes in climate.

References

1. BAHS, 2016. http://dahd.nic.in/Division/statistics/animal-husbandry-statistics-division.
2. Besbes, B. 2009. Genotype evaluation and breeding of poultry for performance under suboptimal village conditions. *World's Poultry Science Journal* **65**: 260-271.
3. Bruford, W. *et al.,* 2003. DNA markers reveal the complexity of livestock domestication. *Nature Review Genetics* **4**: 900-910.
4. Caballero, A. and Toro, M.A. 2002. Analysis of genetic diversity for the management of conserved subdivided populations. *Conservation Genetics* **3**: 289-299.
5. Eding, H. and Bennewitz, J. 2007. Measuring genetic diversity in farm animals. In Oldenbroek K. (Eds). Utilisation and conservation of farm animal genetic resources. Wageningen Academic Publishers, the Netherlands: 103-130.
6. Eding, H. and Meuwissen, T.H.E. 2001. Marker based estimates of between and within population kinships for the conservation of genetic diversity. *Journal of Animal Breeding and Genetics* **118**: 141-159.
7. Eding, H., Crooijmans, R.P.M.A., Groenen, M.A.M. and Meuwissen, T.H.E. 2002. Assessing the contribution of breeds to genetic diversity in conservation schemes. *Genetics Selection Evolution* **34**: 613-634.

8. FAO, 2007. The State of the World's Animal Genetic Resources for Food and Agriculture, edited by B.Rischkowsky and D. Pilling. Rome. http:// www.fao.org/docrep/ 010/ a1250e/ a1250e00.htm.

9. Frankham, R., Ballou, J. and Briscoe, D.A. 2002. Introduction to Conservation Genetics. Cambridge University Press.

10. Granevitze, Z., Hillel, J., Chen, G.H., Cuc, N.T.K., Feldman, M., Eding, H. and Weigend, S. 2007. Genetic diversity within chicken populations from different continents and management histories. *Anim. Genet.* **38**: 576-583.

11. *http://barcoding.si.edu*

12. http://www.nbagr.res.in/regchi.html

13. Muchadeyi, F.C., Eding, H., Simianer, H., Wollny, C.B.A., Groeneveld, E. and Weigend, S. 2008. Mitochondrial DNA D-loop sequences suggest a Southeast Asian and Indian origin of Zimbabwean village chickens. *Anim. Genet.* **39**: 615-622.

14. Oka, T., Ino, Y., Nomura, K., Kawashima, S., Kuwayama, T., Hanada, H., Amano, T., Takada, M., Takahata, N., Hayashi, Y. and Akishinonomiya, F. 2007. Analysis of mtDNA sequences shows Japanese native chicken have multiple origins. *Animal Genetics* **38**: 287-293.

15. Pankaj, P.K., Ramana, D.B.V., M. Nikhila, Rita Rani, D. Sudheer and Choudhary, K.P. 2013 Thermotolerance of sheep in relation to coat colour. *Journal of Agrometeorology* **15:** 163-169.

16. Pinent, T., Simianer, H. and Weigend, S. 2005. Weitzman's approach and conservation of breed diversity: First application to German chicken breeds. Proceeding of the Role of Biotechnology, Rome, Italy. http://www.fao.org/biotech/docs/pinent.pdf

17. Pritchard, J.K., Stephens, M. and Donnerly, P. 2000. Inference of population structure using multicocus genotype data. *Genetics* **155**: 945-959.

18. Reynolds, J., Weir, B.S. and Cockerham, C.C. 1983. Estimation of the coancestry coefficient: Basis for a Short-Term Genetic Distance. *Genetics* **105**: 767-779.

19. Silva, P., Xiaojing Guan, Olivia Ho-Shing, Jess Jones, Jun Xu, Deng Hui, David Notter, and Edward Smith. 2009. Mitochondrial DNA-based Analysis of Genetic Variation and Relatedness among Sri Lankan Indigenous Chickens and the Ceylon Junglefowl (*Gallus lafayetti*). *Anim Genet.* **40(1):** 1-9.

20. Simianer, H. 2005. Decision-making in livestock conservation. *Ecological Economics* **53**: 559-572.

21. Singh, V. (2004) CPR-centred farming in the mountains. Leisa India December, 2004.

22. Tapio, I., Varv, S., Bennewitz, J., Maleviciute, J., Fimland, E., Grislis, Z., Meuwissen, T.H.E., Miceikiene, I., Olsaker, I., Viinalass, H., Vilkki, J. and Kantanen, J. 2006. Prioritization for conservation of northern European cattle breeds based on analysis of microsatellite data. *Conservation Biology* **20**: 1768-1769.

23. Tieu, H.V., Ly, L.V., Sat, L.V. and Su, V.V. 2008. Vietnamese livestock genetic resources conservation and exploitation from 1990 to 2007. Vietnamese J. Anim. Sci. Technol. special volume: 1-10.

24. Weigend, S. and Romanov, M.N. 2001. Current strategies for the assessment and evaluation of genetic diversity in chicken resources. *World's Poultry Science Journal* **57**: 257-288.

25. Weitzman, M.L. 1992. On diversity. *Quarterly Journal of Economics* **CVII**: 363-405.

26. Weitzman, M.L. 1993. What to preserve? An application of diversity theory to crane conservation. *Quarterly Journal of Economics* **CVIII**: 157-183.

□□□

9

Use of Exogenous Fibrolytic Enzymes as Feed Additive in Small Ruminants

G.G. Sheikh*, A.M. Ganai, Tabinda Sehar, Vikas Mahajan and Parvaiz Reshi

* Division of Animal Nutrition, Faculty of Veterinary Sciences and Animal Husbandry, Sher-e-Kashmir University of Agricultural Sciences and Technology of Kashmir Shuhama, Alusteng, Srinagar-190 006, Jammu and Kashmir

Forages are the major component of ruminant rations throughout the production systems in the world. They are consumed by ruminants in a variety of situations, ranging from grazing forages to consumption of processed forage as a component of total mixed diets (Romney & Gill, 2000). Forages, such as straws, are a potential feed for ruminant animals, as ruminants are best adapted to the utilization of plant cell walls (Hungate, 1966) for conversion of fibrous feed sources into milk and meat products. However, the efficiency of utilization of forages for meat and milk production depends on the digestibility of forage cell walls (Beauchemin *et al.*, 2004a).

The use of exogenous enzymes to improve forage utilization and digestibility was first examined for ruminant performance in the 1960's (Burroughs *et al.*, 1960). Unfortunately, many of these early enzyme products were poorly characterized, animal responses were variable, and little or no effort was made to design these products specifically for ruminants. At that time, production of exogenous enzymes was expensive, as fermentation systems were poorly defined and the proper isolates and tools of molecular biology were not available to lower the cost of enzyme production.

a) Method of enzyme treatment and their mode of action

Enzymes have been applied to TMR (Higginbotham *et al.*, 1996; Beauchemin *et al.*, 1999; Phipps *et al.*, 2000; Yang *et al.*, 2000; Thakur *et al.*, 2008), hay (Beauchemin *et al.*, 1995; Lewis *et al.*, 1996; Yang *et al.*, 1999), ensiled forages (Beauchemin *et al.*, 1995), concentrate (Rode *et al.*, 1999; Phipps *et al.*, 2000; Yang *et al.*, 2000), supplement (Bowman, 2001), or premix (Bowman, 2001). Applying brolytic exogenous enzymes in a liquid form onto feeds prior to consumption can have a positive effect on animal performance (Kung *et al.*, 2000; Yang *et al.*, 2000). Exogenous enzymes may be expected to be more effective, when applied to high moisture feeds (such as silages) compared to dry feeds because of the higher moisture content. The requirement for water in the hydrolysis of soluble sugars from complex polymers is a fundamental biochemical principle. Furthermore, silage pH values are usually at, or around, the optimal pH for most fungal enzymes. However, in practice, some exogenous enzymes are more effective, when applied in a liquid form to dry forage as opposed to wet forage.

b) Mode of action: An integrated hypothesis

Beauchemin and Holtshausen (2010) argued that the mode of action of exogenous enzymes is still relatively unknown, due to the complex nature of the ruminal microbial ecosystem and the process of fibre digestion. However, lack of understanding of the mode of action of exogenous enzymes could be categorised under pre-ruminal or pre-consumption, ruminal, and post-ruminal effects (Meale *et al.*, 2014). Application of exogenous enzymes onto forages or to the diets of ruminants before consumption can initiate fibre hydrolysis through DM loss (Krueger *et al.*, 2008). Exogenous fibrolytic enzymes applied to feed before consumption bind to the feed and this makes them more active in the rumen, possibly because of their increased resistance to proteolysis and outflow of ruminal content, thus prolonging their residence time in the rumen. (Beauchemin *et al.*, 2003) showed that enzymatic activities declined when two different EFE products, where administered directly into the rumen due to enzyme inactivation and passage of fluid from the rumen. Similarly, maximizing the proportion of the diet to which the enzyme is added is considered to increase the chances that the enzymes will remain active in the rumen.

Most of the improvements in forage quality resulting from exogenous enzymes application were previously attributed to ruminal effects (Beauchemin *et al.*, 2003). Supplementing ruminant diets with exogenous enzymes increases the rate but seldom the extent of feed digestion (Krueger *et al.*, 2008). Therefore, Meale *et al.* (2014) suggested that the positive responses from exogenous enzymes are not a result of these preparations solubilizing substrates; rather, an increase in total enzymatic activity in the rumen can increase ruminal hydrolytic capacity, which can enhance the digestibility of the complete diet. As such, digestibility of both non-fibrous and fibrous fractions can increase; explaining why exogenous enzymes can also be effective in increasing the digestibility of non-fibre fractions in high concentrate diets (Arriola and Adesogan, 2013). A synergistic relationship between exogenous enzymes and rumen microbiota, and an increase in bacterial attachment are other likely modes of action of exogenous enzymes in the rumen (Meale *et al.*, 2014). Giraldo *et al.* (2008, 2009) showed that exogenous enzymes increased microbial growth and production of microbial protein. Furthermore, Morgavi *et al.* (2000) in early study showed that synergism acts to increase the effects of both indigenous ruminal microbes and exogenous enzymes so that the combined response exceeds the additive effects of each individual component. However, increased amounts of exogenous enzymes can also compete with the ruminal microbial populations for cellulose binding sites on feed, potentially explaining the lack of or even negative responses observed with the increased amounts of exogenous enzyme supplementation *in-vivo*. For exogenous enzymes to be effective, it is important that they complement and not replace the existing natural enzyme activities produced by ruminal microbes (Meale *et al.*, 2014). Adding exogenous fibrolytic enzymes to ruminant diets can also impact nutrient digestion in the hindgut.

Hristov *et al.* (1998a) reported that approximately 30 and 5% of xylanases and endoglucanase, respectively, can escape ruminal fermentation and are active in intestinal digesta of ruminants. Depending on application level, other fibrolytic enzymes may also bypass the rumen and increase polysaccharide-degrading activities in intestinal digesta (Chesson, 1994). This along with other reports (Fontes *et al.*, 1995; Morgavi *et al.*, 2001) seems to indicate that xylanases are more resistant to ruminal and abomasal conditions than endoglucanases. Presently, although post-ruminal effects can be documented, they are thought to account for a minor component of any positive responses observed with existing enzyme preparations, with improvements primarily arising from positive alterations in rumen function (Meale *et al.*, 2014). However, to date, no studies have directly quantified the relative importance of fibrolytic enzymes by pre-consumption, ruminal or post-ruminal action either on animal performance or feed digestibility.

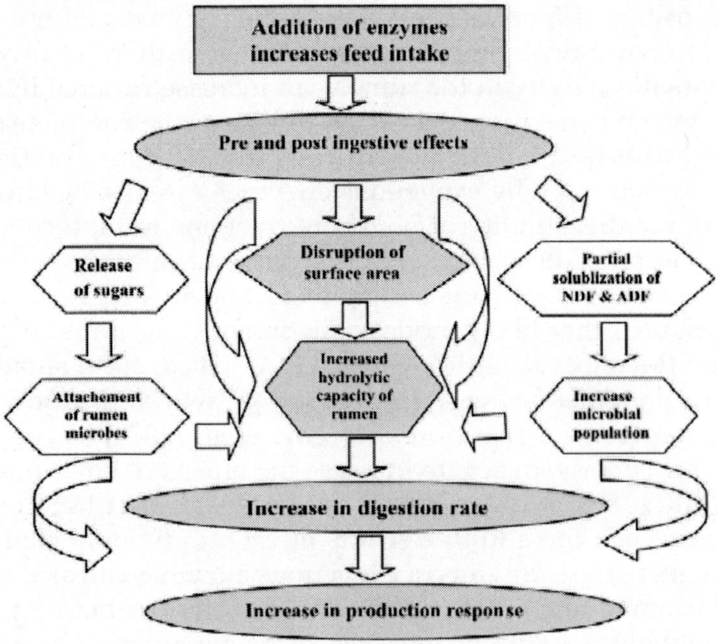

Fig. 3: A general scheme representation to explain mode of action of fibrolytic enzymes

c) Effect on growth and nutrient utilization

Final assessment of the true value of exogenous enzymes for ruminants in terms of improving feed utilization can only be accessed through the use of animal production trials. A variety of effects of using cell wall degrading enzymes in ruminant diets has been reported in past and recent studies. Different domestic ruminants at various stages of production have been used. Various types of forages have been fed, and the enzyme products in those studies were given to the animals in diverse ways at the time of feeding; sprayed onto forage, added to concentrate, sprayed onto the total mixed ration (TMR), added as dry powder to feed, or ruminally infused (Beauchemin and Holtshausen, 2010).

Enzyme supplementation is often accompanied by increased feed intake (Gado and Salem, 2008; Gado *et al.*, 2007, 2009) which may partly be due to increased palatability of the diet due to sugars released by pre-ingestive fibre hydrolysis. However, post-ingestive enzyme effects, such as increased digestion rate and/or extent of digestion (Beauchemin and Rode, 1996; Feng *et al.*, 1996; Gado and Salem, 2008; Titi, 2004; Krueger *et al.*, 2008) may increase hydrolytic activity in the rumen to reduce gut fill and enhance feed intake (Arriola and Adesogan, 2013). Ganai (2011) also found that supplementation of feed with enzymes alone and in mixture with probiotics and herbs improve feed intake, body weight gain, feed efficiency and nutrient digestibility in kids. In support Arce-Cervantes *et al.* (2013) and Saleem *et al.* (2011) found improved the cellulolytic activity in the rumen fluid of lambs fed fibrolytic enzymes, thereby increasing DM intake, feed efficiency as well as the digestibility and body weight gain. Fibrolytic enzymes have improved intake, digestibility, feed efficiency, growth and productive performance of lambs (Arce-Cervantes *et al.,* 2013). Similarly, Gado *et al.* (2011) found Ossimi male lambs fed paddy straw ensiled orange pulp treated with exogenous enzymes highest average daily gain (ADG) than control. This trend was consistent with the results of Bassiouni *et al.* (2011) and Khattab *et al.* (2013) who also found similar effect of fibrolytic enzymes supplementation on *In Situ* degradability of DM, CP and CF of different rations consisted of concentrate and rice straw. Treatment of rice straw with exogenous enzymes reported increased ($P<0.01$) the degradation of NDF and ADF (Gado *et al.*, 2013 and Diaz *et al.*, 2013). The results are consistent with reports of other researchers (Giraldo *et al.*, 2014; Dean *et al.*, 2013; Mendoza *et al.*, 2013;Tang *et al.*, 2013; Arriola *et al.*, 2011; Ganai *et al.*, 2011; Saleem *et al.*, 2011; Das and Singh, 2010; Gado *et al.*, 2009; Gado and Salem, 2008; Singh and Das, 2008, 2009 a, b; Kaur *et al.*, 2007; Miachieo and Thakur, 2007) reported increased nutrient digestibility on supplementation of fibrolytic enzymes in diets of sheep. In a recent study Thammiaha *et al.* (2016) reported improved IVDMD of different crop residues by lignin peroxidases obtained from white rot fungi with decreased NDF, ADF and lignin of all the treated straw compared to the untreated control straws.

On the other hand, only marginal improvement or no effect on DMI has also been reported by enzyme supplementation or enzyme treatment (Titi and Lubbadeh 2004; Muwalla *et al.*, 2007; Miller *et al.*, 2008, Singh and Das, 2008, 2009a; Das and Singh 2010; Dean *et al.* 2013; Mendoza *et al.*, 2013; Torres *et al.*, 2013). Generally, the application of exogenous enzymes to the diets of small ruminants has had little impact on feed intake and production performance; therefore, most research work in this area has focused on digestibility studies (Meale *et al.*, 2014). Some other studies have also reported no effect on nutrient digestibility with the use of exogenous fibrolytic enzymes (Bueno *et al.*, 2013; Torres *et al.*, 2013; Vargas *et al.*, 2013; Awawdeh and

Obeidat, 2011; Giraldo *et al.*, 2008; Muwalla *et al.*, 2007; Knowlton *et al.*, 2002; Yang *et al.*, 2000). Similarly, Giraldo *et al.* (2008) inoculated exogenous fibrolytic enzymes (12 g/lamb daily; Fibrozyme; Alltech Inc.) directly into the rumen of fistulated Merino sheep before feeding a grass hay concentrate diet (70:30; DM basis) and reported no effect on diet digestibility. No effect was observed on DMI, ADG, feed conversion, or wool growth in Dorset-cross ewe lambs fed barley based diet treated with a commercial exogenous enzyme (Miller *et al.*, 2008). Additionally, Rojo *et al.* (2005) fed exogenous amylases from *B. licheniformis* and *A. niger* (up to 2.90 g enzyme/kg DM sorghum) and observed no effects on production performance in Suffolk lambs. Wang and Xue (2016) also reported no effect of cellulose supplementation on nutrient digestibility, energy utilization and methane emission by Boer crossbred goats. These variations in nutrient digestibility, observed by the addition of fibrolytic enzymes may be due to many factors, such as forage level, enzyme level, ruminal pH, rumen retention time and method of enzyme application (Colombatto *et al.*, 2003). The higher the forage level, the more likely to observe a positive response on performance (Vicini *et al.*, 2003; Ranilla *et al.*, 2008).

d) Effect of fibrolytic enzymes on wool parameters

Apart from level of nutrition the other components affecting efficiency of wool production are digestibility of diet, body weight, season (Butler and Maxwell, 1984) and the metabolic efficiency of the individual animals (Kott *et al.*, 1999). The changes in wool growth and characteristics are associated with quality and relative mixture of absorbed amino acids even at the same dry matter intake (Ferguson, 1967). Jafari *et al.* (2005) reported treated wheat straw with exogenous fiber-degrading enzymes @ 10, 20 and 30% as replacement for alfalfa hay in Naieni breed ewe lambs had no effect on final fleece weight, and fleece weight index, wool production per day, feed conversion to wool, final staple length, wool and hair crimp per centimeter of length, per cent of heterotype, coronal, kemp, reticulate and imbricate fibres and accumulation of scales in 100 μm fibre lengths. However, feeding untreated wheat straw tended to decrease final fleece weight, wool production, and final staple length. According to Nsereko *et al.* (2002) adding feed enzymes to the diets directly, increased the numbers of non-fibrolytic, as well as fibrolytic bacteria in the rumen. The stimulation on wool growth rate resulting from treating wheat straw with feed enzymes can be explained by an increased growth of reticuloruminal micro-organisms and microbial flow to the small intestine, hence a greater absorption of amino acids and supply of metabolizable protein to the animal. Similarly, Hoaglund *et al.* (1992) reported that feeding untreated wheat straw tended to decrease final fleece weight, wool production, and numerically increased final wool diameter.

References

1. Arce-Cervantes,O., Mendoza, G.D., Hernández, P.A., Meneses, M., Torres-Salado,N. and Loera,O. 2013.The Effects of a lignocellulolytic extract of fomes sp. EUM1 on the intake, digestibility, feed efficiency and growth of lambs. *Animal Nutrition and Feed Technology* **13**: 363-372.
2. Arriola, K.G. and Adesogan, A.T. 2013. Effect of fibrolytic enzyme application on the digestibility of corn silage, alfalfa hay, concentrates, and complete diets under simulated ruminal and preruminal conditions. *Animal Feed Science and Technology* **13**: 537-550.
3. Arriola, K.G., Kim, S.C., Staples, C.R. and Adesogan, A.T. 2011. Effect of fibrolytic enzyme application to low and high-concentrate diets on the performance of lactating dairy cattle. *Journal of Dairy Science* **94**: 832-841.
4. Awawdeh, M.S. and Obeidat, B.S. 2011. Effect of supplemental exogenous enzymes on performance of finishing Awassi lambs fed olive cake-containing diets. *Livestock Science* **138**: 20-24.
5. Bassiouni, M.I., Gaafar, H.M.A., Mohi, A.A.A., El-Din, Metwally, A.M. and Elshora, M.A.H. 2011. Evaluation of rations supplemented with fibrolytic enzyme on dairy cows performance 2. *In situ* ruminal degradability of rations containing different roughages at two concentrate to roughage ratios. *Researcher* **3**: 21-33.
6. Beauchemin, K.A. and Holtshausen, L. 2010. Developments in enzyme usage in ruminants. **In**: *Enzymes in Farm Animal Nutrition,* 2nd ed. (Eds. M.R. Bedford and G.G. Partridge), CABI, Oxford, United Kingdom, pp. 206-230.
7. Beauchemin, K.A. and Rode L.M. 1996. Use of feed enzymes in ruminant nutrition. **In**: *Proceeding of Canadian Society of Animal Science* (Ed. Rode L.M.), Lethbridge, AB, Canada, pp. 103-130.
8. Beauchemin, K.A., Colombatto, D. and Morgavi, D.P. 2004. A rationale for the development of feed enzyme products for ruminants. *Canadian Journal of Animal Science* **84**: 23-36.

9. Beauchemin, K.A., Colombatto, D., Morgavi, D.P. and Yang, W.Z. 2003. Use of exogenous fibrolytic enzymes to improve feed utilization by ruminants. *Journal of Animal Science* **81**: E37-E47.
10. Beauchemin, K.A., Rode, L.M. and Sewaltm, V. J. H. (1995). Fibrolytic enzymes increase digestibility and growth rate of steers fed dry forage. *Canadian Journal of Animal Science* **75**: 641-644.
11. Beauchemin, K.A., Rode, L.M. and Karren, D. 1999. Use of feed enzymes in feedlot finishing diets. *Canadian. Journal of Animal Science* **79**: 243-246.
12. Bowman, G.R., Beauchemin, K.A. and Shelford, J.A. 2002. The proportion of the diet to which fibrolytic enzymes are added affects nutrient digestion by lactating dairy cows. *Journal of Dairy Science* **85**: 3420-3429.
13. Bueno, A.L., Mendoza Martínez, G.D., Hernández García, P.A., Martínez García, J.A. and Plata Pérez, F.X. 2013. Evaluation of high doses of exogenous fibrolytic enzymes in lambs fed an oat straw based ration. *Animal Feed Science Technology* **13**: 355-362.
14. Burroughs, W., Woods, W., Ewing, S. A., Greig, J. and Theurer, B. 1960. Enzyme additions to fattening cattle rations. *Journal of Animal Science* **19**: 458-464.
15. Butler, L.G. and Maxwell, M.M.C. 1984. A review of efficiency of conversion of feed into wool. *Animal Breeding Abstracts* **52**:475-485.
16. Chesson, L. 1994. Manipulation of fibre degradation: an old theme revisited. Pages 83-98.
17. Colombatto, D., Mould, F.L., Bhat, M.K. and Owen, E. 2003. Use of fibrolytic enzymes to improve the nutritive value of ruminant diets. *Animal Feed Science and Technology* **107**: 201-209.
18. Das, M.M. and Singh, K.K. 2010.Effect of fibrolytic enzyme treatment of ammoniated sorghum stover on nutrient intake and utilization in calves. *Indian Veterinary Journal* **87**: 687-688.
19. Dean D.B., Staples, C.R., Littell, R.C., Kim,S. and Adesogan, A.T. 2013.Effect of method of adding a fibrolytic enzyme to dairy cow diets on feed intake digestibility, milk production, ruminal fermentation, and blood metabolites. *Animal Feed Science and Technology* **13**: 337-353.
20. Díaz, A., Carro, M.D., Saro, C., Mateos, I., Odongo, E. and Ranilla, M.J. 2013. *In vitro* evaluation of commercial fibrolytic enzymes for improving the nutritive value of low-quality forages. *Animal Nutrition and Feed Technology* **13**: 461-476.

21. Feng, P., Hunt, C.W., Pritchard, G.T. and Julien, W.E. 1996. Effect of enzyme preparations on *in situ* and *in-vitro* degradation and *in vivo* digestive characteristics of mature cool-season grass forage in beef steers. *Journal of Animal Science* **74**: 1349-1357.

22. Ferguson, K.A., Hemsley J.A. and Reis, P.J. 1967. Nutrition and wool growth. The effect of protecting dietary protein from microbial degradation in the rumen. *Asian-Australasian Journal of Animal Science* **30**: 215-217.

23. Fontes, C.M.G.A., Hall, J., Hirst, B.H., Hazlewood, G.P. and Gilbert, H.J. 1995. The resistance of cellulases and xylanases to proteolytic inactivation. *Applied Microbiology and Biotechnology* **43**: 52-57.

24. Gado, H.M., Salem, A.Z.M., Camacho, L.M., Elghandour, M.M.Y. and Salazar, M.C. 2013. Influence of exogenous enzymes on *in-vitro* ruminal degradation of ensiled rice straw with DDGS. *Animal Nutrition and Feed Technology* **13**: 569-574.

25. Gado, H.M., Salem, A.Z.M., Odongo, N.E. and Borhami, B.E. 2011. Influence of exogenous enzymes ensiled with orange pulp on digestion and growth performance in lambs. *Animal Nutrition and Feed Technology* **165**: 131-136.

26. Gado, H.M. and Salem, A.Z.M. 2008. Influence of exogenous enzymes from anaerobic source on growth performance, digestibility, ruminal fermentation and blood metabolites in lambs fed of orange pulp silage in total mixed ration. **In**: *59th Annual Meeting of the European Association for Animal Production,* Vilnius, Lithuania, August 24-27, pp. 228.

27. Gado, H.M., Salem, A.Z.M., Robinson, P.H. and Hassan, M. 2009. Influence of exogenous enzymes on nutrient digestibility, extent of ruminal fermentation as well as milk production and composition in dairy cows. *Animal Feed Science Technology* **154**: 36-46.

28. Gado, H.M.., Meiwally, H.M. Soliman, H., Basiony, A.Z.L. and El Gahil, E.R. 2007. Enzymatic treatments of bagasse by different sources of cellulase enzymes. **In**: *The 11th Conf. Animal Nutr., Al-Aqsor-Aswan,* Egypt November, 13-18, vol. 10, Pp. 607.

29. Ganai, A.M. 2011. Effect of various feed additives alone and in combination on nutrient utilization and growth performance in goats. PhD thesis, Swami Keshwanand Rajasthan Agriculture University, Bikaner.

30. Giraldo, L.A., Tejido, M.L., Ranilla, M.J., Ramos, S. and Carro, M.D. 2008. Influence of direct fed Fibrolytic enzymes on diet digestibility

and ruminal activity in sheep fed grass hay based diet. *Journal of Animal Science* **86**: 1617-1623.

31. Giraldo, L.A., Tejido, M.L., Ranilla, M.J., Ramos, S., Mantecon, A.R. and Carro, M.D. 2009. Influence of direct fed exogenous fibrolytic enzymes on ruminal fibrolytic activity in sheep. *Options Mediterraneennes* **85**: 297-302.

32. Giraldo, L.A., Tejido, M.L., Ranilla, M.J., Ramos S. and Carro, M.D. 2014. Influence of direct-fed fibrolytic enzymes on diet digestibility and ruminal activity in sheep fed a grass hay-based diet. *Journal of Animal Science* **86**: 1617-1623.

33. Higginbotham, G.E., dePetters, E.J., Berry, S.L. and Ahmadi, A. 1996. Effect of adding a cell wall degrading enzyme to a total mixed ration for lactating dairy cows. *Professional Animal Scientist* **12**: 81-85.

34. Hoaglund, C.M., Thomas, V.M., Petersen, M.K. and Kott, R.W. 1992. Effects of supplemental protein source and metabolizable energy intake on nutritional status in pregnant ewes. *Journal of Animal Science* **70**: 273-280.

35. Hristov, A.N., McAllister, T.A. and Cheng, K.J. 1998. Effect of dietary or abomasal supplementation of exogenous polysaccharide-degrading enzymes on rumen fermentation and nutrient digestibility. *Journal of Animal Science* **76**: 3146-3156.

36. Hungate, R. E. 1966. The rumen and its microbes. Academic Press, New York.

37. Jafari A., Edriss, M.A., Alikhani, M. and Emtiazi, G. 2005. Effects of treated wheat straw with exogenous fibre-degrading enzymes on wool characteristics of ewe lambs. *Pakistan Journal of Nutrition* **4**(5): 321-326.

38. Kaur, P., Palaha, R., Sareen, V.K. and Singh, S. 2007. Effect of fibrozyme supplementation of rumen metabolism and nutrient digestibility in buffalo calves. *Indian Journal of Animal Science* **24**: 62-64.

39. Khattab, H.M., Gado, H.M., Salem, A.Z.M., Camacho, L.M., El-Sayed, M.M., Kholif, A.M., El-Shewy, A.A. and Kholif, A.E. 2013. Chemical composition and *in-vitro* digestibility of *Pleurotus ostreatus* spent rice straw. *Animal Nutriion and Feed Technology* **13**: 507-516.

40. Knowlton, K.F., McKinney, J.M., and Cobb, C. 2002. Effect of a direct-fed fibrolytic enzyme formulation on nutrient intake,

partitioning, and excretion in early and late lactation Holstein cows. *Journal of Dairy Science* **85**: 3328-3335.

41. Kott, R., Hatfield P. and Schuldt, M. 1999. Wool VS. Lamb production. SDSU Sheep Day and USSSA Regional Workshop. Brookings, SD, USA.

42. Krueger, N.A. and Adesogan, A.T. 2008. Effects of different mixtures of fibrolytic enzymes on digestion and fermentation and fermentation of bahiagrass hay. *Animal Feed Science and Technology* **145**: 84-94.

43. Kung, J.L., Treacher, R.J., Nauman, G.A., Smagala, A.M., Endres, K.M. and Cohen, M.A. 2000. The effect of treating forages with fibrolytic enzymes on its nutritive value and lactation performance of dairy cows. *Journal of Dairy Science* **83**: 115-122.

44. Lewis, G.E., Hunt, C.W., Sanchez, W.K., Treacher, R., Pritchard, G.T. and Feng, P. 1996. Effect of direct-fed fibrolytic enzymes on the digestive characteristics of a forage based diet fed to beef steers. *Journal of Animal Science* **74**: 3020-3028.

45. Meale, S.J., Beauchemin, K.A., Hristov, A.N., Chaves, A.V. and McAllister, T.A. 2014. BoardInvited Review: Opportunities and challenges in using exogenous enzymes to improve ruminant production. *Journal of Animal Science* **92**: 427-442.

46. Mendoza, G.D., Mota, N., Plata, F.X., Martinez, J.A. and Hernández, P.A. 2013. Effects of exogenous glucoamylase from aspergillusniger and grain level on performance of the lambs. *Animal Nutriion and Feed Technology* **13**: 391-398.

47. Miachieo, K. and Thakur, S.S. 2007. Effect of exogenous fibrolytic enzymes on the productive performance of lactating Sahiwal cows. *Indian Journal of Animal Nutrition* **24**: 27-30.

48. Miller, D.R., Elliott, R. and Norton, B.W. 2008. Effects of an exogenous enzyme, Roxazyme® G2 Liquid, on digestion and utilisation of barley and sorghum grain-based diets by ewe lambs. *Animal Feed Science and Technology* **140**: 90-109.

49. Morgavi, D.P., Beauchemin, K.A., Nsereko, V.L., Rode, L.M., Iwaasa, A.D., Yang, W.Z., McAllister, T.A. and Wang, Y. 2000. Synergy between ruminal fibrolytic enzymes and enzymes from *Trichoderma longibrachiatum*. *Journal of Dairy Science* **83**: 1310-1321.

50. Morgavi, D.P., Beauchemin, K.A., Nsereko, V.L., Rode, L.M., McAllister, T.A., Iwaasa, A.D., Wang, Y. and Yang, W.Z. 2001. Resistance of feed enzymes to proteolytic inactivation by rumen

micro-organisms and gastro-intestinal proteases. *Journal of Animal Science* **79**: 1621-1630.

51. Muwalla, M.M., Hadddad, S.G. and Hijajeen, M.A. 2007. Effect of fibrolytic enzyme inclusion in high concentrate fattening diets on nutrient digestibility and growth performance of Awassi lambs. *Livestock Sci.* **111**: 255-258.

52. Nsereko, V.L., Beauchemin, K.A., Morgavi, D.P., Rode, L.M., Furtado, A.F., McAllister, T.A., Iwaasa, A.D., Yang, W.Z. and Wang, Y. 2002. Effect of a fibrolytic enzyme preparation from *Trichoderma longibrachiatum* on the rumen microbial population of dairy cows. *Canadian Journal of Microbiology* **48**: 14-20.

53. Phipps, R.H., Sutton, J.D., Beever, D.E., Bhat, M.K., Hartnell, G.F., Vicini, J. and Hard, D.L. 2000. Effect of cell-wall degrading enzymes and method of application on feed intake and milk production of Holstein-Friesian dairy cows. *Journal of Dairy Science* **83**(Suppl. 1): 236-237 (Abstr.).

54. Ranilla, M.J., Tejido, M.L., Giraldo, L.A., Tricarico, J.M. and Carro, M.D. 2008. Effects of an exogenous fibrolytic enzyme preparation on *in vitro* ruminal fermentation of three forages and their isolated cell walls. *Animal Feed Science and Technology* **145**: 109-121.

55. Rode, L.M., Yang, W.Z. and Beauchemin, K.A. 1999. Fibrolytic enzyme supplementation for dairy cows in early lactation. *Journal of Dairy Science* **82**: 2121-2126.

56. Rojo, R., Mendoza, G.D., Gonz´alez, S.S., Landois, L., B´arcena, R. and Crosby, M.M. 2005. Effects of exogenous amylases from *Bacillus licheniformis* and *Aspergillus niger* on ruminal starch digestion and lamb performance. *Animal Feed Science and Technology* **124**: 655-665.

57. Saleem, A.Z.M., El-Adawy, M.M., Gado, H., Camacho, L.M., González-Ronquillo, M., Alsersy, H. and Borhami, B. 2011. Effects of exogenous enzymes on nutrients digestibility and growth performance in sheep and goats. *Tropical and Subtropical Agroecosystems* **14**: 867-874.

58. Singh, K.K and Das, M.M. 2009a. Effect of fibrolytic enzyme treated roughage on nutrient utilization and growth performance in kids. *Indian Journal of Animal Science* **79(6):** 620-622.

59. Singh, K.K and Das, M.M. 2009b. Effect of fibrolytic enzyme treated wheat straw on rumen fermentation and nutrient utilization in calves. *Indian Veterinary Journal* **86**: 380-382.

60. Singh, K.K. and Das, M.M. 2008. Effect of fibrolytic enzymes treatment of oat hay on rumen fermentation and nutrient utilization in goats. *Indian Veterinary Journal* **85**: 1070-1072.

61. Tang S.X., Zou, Y., Wang, M., Salem, A.Z.M., Odongo, N.E., Zhou, C.S., Han, X.F., Tan, Z.L., Zhang, M., Fu, Y.F., Huang, S.Q., He, Z.X. and Kang, J.H. 2013. Effects of exogenous cellulase source on *in-vitro* fermentation characteristics and methane production of crop straws and grasses. *Animal Nutriion and Feed Technology* **13**: 489-505.

62. Thakur, S.S., Tomar, S.K. and Sirohi, S.K. 2008. *In vitro* DM and cell wall degradability of total mixed rations influenced by exogenous fibrolytic enzyme supplementation. *Indian Journal of Animal Nutrition* **25**(3): 219-223.

63. Thammiaha, V., Ramya, G. Rao., Samaanta, A.K., Senani S. and Sridhar, M. 2016. *In-vitro* efficacy of lignin peroxidases obtained from white rot fungi in enhancing the digestibility of crop residues for feeding ruminants. **In**: *Proc. of XVI Biennial Animal Nutrition Conference on Innovative Approaches for Animal Feeding and Nutrition Research,* February 6-8, 2016 NDRI, Karnal, pp.23.

64. Titi, H. 2004. Response of Awassi lambs to enzymic treatment fed two different forages. 1: Digestibility and growth performance. *Dirasat. Agricultural Science* **31**: 302-310.

65. Titi, H. and Lubbadeh, W.F. 2004. Effect of feeding cellulase enzyme on productive responses of pregnant and lactating ewes and goats. *Small Ruminant Research* **52**: 137-143.

66. Torres, N., Mendoza, G.D., Bárcena, R., Loera, O., González, S., Aranda, E., Hernández, P.A. and Crosby M. 2013. Effects of various fibrolytic enzyme extracts on digestibility and productive performance of lambs fed a forage-based diet. *Animal Nutriion and Feed Technology* **13**: 381-389.

67. Vargas, J.M., Mendoza, G.D., De la Salud Rubio-Lozano, M. and Castrejón, F.A. 2013. Effect of exogenous fibrolytic enzymes on the carcass characteristics and performance of grain-finished steers. *Animal Feed Science and Technology* **13**: 435-439.

68. Vicini, J.L., Bateman, H.G, Bhat, M.K., Clark, J.H., Erdman, R.A., Phipps, R.H., Amburgh, M.E., Hartnell, G.F., Hintz, R.L. and Hard, D.L. 2003. Effect of feeding supplemental fibrolytic enzymes or soluble sugars with malic acid on milk production. *Journal of Dairy Science* **86**: 576-585.

69. Wang, L. and Xue B. 2016. Effects of cellulase supplementation on nutrient digestibility, energy utilization and methane emission by Boer crossbred goats. *Asian-Australasian Journal of Animal Science* **29**(2): 204-210.

70. Yang, W.Z., Beauchemin, K.A. and Rode, L.M. 1999. Effects of an enzyme feed additive on extent of digestion and milk production in lactating dairy cows. *Journal of Dairy Science* **82**: 391-403.

71. Yang, W.Z., Beauchemin, K.A. and Rode, L.M. 2000. A comparison of methods of adding fibrolytic enzymes to lactating cow diets. *Journal of Dairy Science* **83(11):** 2512-2520.

□□□

10

Concept and Use of Complete Feed System in Small Ruminants

G.G. Sheikh*, A.M. Ganai, Tabinda Sehar, Vikas Mahajan and Ishfaq Ahmad

* Division of Animal Nutrition, Faculty of Veterinary Sciences and Animal Husbandry, Sher-e-Kashmir University of Agricultural Sciences and Technology of Kashmir Shuhama, Alusteng, Srinagar-190 006, Jammu and Kashmir

Complete feed or total mixed ration being a quantitative mixture of all dietary ingredients, provide the specific nutrients requirements. In this system the animals have continuous free choice availability of a uniform feed mixture resulting in more uniform load on the rumen (Lailer *et al.*, 2005). The basic principle of complete feed system is that all the feed ingredients inclusive of roughages and concentrates are mixed together to form a uniform mixture, ensuring a synchronous and proportionate supply of essential nutrients in the diet.

Complete feed for better utilization of crop residues

Concept of complete feed with the use of poor crop residues is a novel way to increase the intake and improve the feed utilization. According to an estimate by Ramachandra *et al.* (2007), these crop residues will provide more than 70% of the feed resources for Indian livestock by the year 2020. These crop residues are poor in palatability and nutritive value, which can be overcome by incorporating in complete rations for ruminants. Further, complete feed improves the feeding value of a poor quality crop residue by ensuring their better utilization, simplifies feeding, controls ratio of roughage to concentrate, provides uniform feed intake, reduces the feed wastage and cost of feeding and avoids refusal of non-palatable portion of plant residues (Ganai *et al.*, 2007). Kishore *et al.*, (2013) stated that feeding of crop residue based complete rations improved nutrient utilization in buffalo bulls when compared to conventional system of feeding. In an another study the author studied the effect of feeding crop residue based complete ration on nutrient utilization in Nellore rams and concluded that complete rations containing crop residues provide better nutrient supply to rams compared to conventional ration (Kishore *et al.,* 2014). Cereal crop residues could be effectively used as roughage source at 50 per cent level in complete rations for the feeding of ram lambs to obtain optimum gain (Malisetty *et al.,* 2013). In complete rations with R:C ratio of 60:40 for sheep, concentrate mixture could be efficiently replaced by leaf meal with no adverse effect on nutrient utilization and better results could be obtained at 30 per cent replacement level (Afzal *et al.,* 2009).

The merit of complete feed also lies in providing stable rumen environment, reduced fermentation losses and less fluctuation in release of ammonia (Lailer *et al.,* 2005). The research works regarding concept and usefulness of complete rations have been extensively discussed throughout the world by numerous workers and was proposed that this feeding method may be used to induce animals to consume roughage and concentrate in proper proportion as well as to achieve better feed utilization, production and to avoid refusal of unpalatable nutrients. Prasad *et al.* (2000) and Singh and Sankhyan (2003) suggested 60% level as to be the optimum level of incorporation of roughage source i.e. groundnut haulms/straw in complete feed for growing lambs. Bhatia *et al.* (2004) reported that blending of roughage and concentrate in the form of complete ration has the beneficial effect in terms of utilization of low grade roughages in Marwari sheep. It increases the voluntary feed intake and ensures efficient utilization of the feed.

Complete feed for better dry matter intake, nutrient digestibility and growth

Complete feed ensures better consumption, avoids refusal of unpalatable nutrients, reduces eating and rumination time and thus, increases resting time. Increased intake of dry matter and nutrients on complete feed system compared to conventional feeding system has been reported by several workers (Verma *et al.,* 2001; Reddy and Reddy, 1998; Reddy *et al.,* 2002; Kirubanath *et al.,* 2003; Waje *et al.,* 2010; Kishore *et al.,* 2014). Blending of roughage and concentrate portions to form a complete ration has beneficial effects in terms of utilization of low-grade roughages; besides, extrusion of the complete mash feed into pellets using expander-extruder (Reddy and Reddy, 1998; Kirubanath *et al.*, 2003; Waje *et al.*, 2010) or its densification into feed blocks (Ganai *et al.*, 2007; Afzal *et al.*, 2009) distinctly improve the nutritive value of mash diet. It increases the voluntary feed intake and ensures efficient utilization of the feed (Bhatia, 2004). Dhuria *et al.*, (2007a) evaluated three iso-nitrogenous complete feeds containing mustard straw at 40, 50 and 60 per cent levels in sheep and concluded from the study that mustard straw can be incorporated in the complete feed upto 60% level without adverse effect on voluntary feed intake and utilization of nutrients in sheep. Waje *et al.*, (2010) reported higher intake and digestibility of nutrients in growing crossbred calves fed mixed forest grasses based complete pelleted feed as compared to calves fed either conventional or TMR diets. A study conducted by Chaturvedi *et al.*, (2009) on two feeding systems, *viz.*, stall feeding (SF) with complete feed and grazing plus supplementation (GR) evaluating body weight gain, nutrient utilization and feed cost of production of Avikalin lambs. The stall feeding system of feeding where complete feed was offered to lambs appeared superior in terms of intake and animal performance. Therefore, the stall feeding system can be advocated as an alternative to grazing and supplementation feeding strategy for sheep production, especially where the pastures are highly eroded and need resting for regeneration or curing.

Complete feed as Feed blocks

Complete feed block is a recent and noble way for incorporation of these feed residues in complete feed. Saina and Patel (2016) reported that under traditional grazing system of rearing the actual growth potential of lambs cannot be achieved. So, balanced feeding in the form of feed block maximizes growth of Magra lambs in arid region. Under temperate conditions Afzal *et al.*, (2009) conducted an experiment on Corriedale lambs fed a complete feed (60:40, R:C. ratio) either in block or mash form for 90 days and reported higher ADG and nitrogen in block fed lambs by 47g/day or 32.2% and 3.0 or 24.0% respectively. However, DM and nutrient intake, FCR and digestibility of DM and gross nutrients, nutritive value and retention of minerals did not change between block or mash fed groups. In support to this Mishra *et al.*, (2013) evaluate the effect of fallen tree leaves (FTL) inclusion (100, 200 and 300 g/kg diet) in high roughage feed block of Malpura rams to utilize forest wastes and concluded that under feed scarcity periods, FTL can safely be used up to 20% level as a roughage component of complete feed block diets. The complete diet based on paddy straw incorporated at 50 per cent level could meet the maintenance requirements in sheep and was more palatable when it was expander extruder pelleted and such processing improved the nutritive value of the diet. Densification of the complete diet had no effect on nutrient digestibility and rumen fermentation pattern in sheep (Nagalakshmi and Reddy, 2012). Kumar *et al.,* (2014) carried out a study to identify appropriate processing method for efficient utilization of sweet sorghum bagasse after blending with concentrate at 50:50 ratio in complete diet for growing lambs and concluded that expander extruded pellet diet was better utilized in terms of nutrient utilization and microbial N supply than chopped or mash form by the growing ram lambs.

Feeding of compete feed can also be adopted under adverse situations, such as drought and famine, which are common phenomenon in arid and semi-arid regions. Dhuria *et al.,* (2010) also reported no adverse effects on rumen fermentation pattern and haematobiochemical parameters in sheep fed bajra straw based complete feed at 60% level in mash and block form. In an another study, Dhuria *et al.,* (2011) fed mustard straw at 60% level in complete feed in mash and block form to growing Magra sheep and reported no adverse effect on rumen fermentation pattern and haemato-biochemical parameters. The use of feed additives in complete feed manipulates rumen environment for better utilization of these low quality crop residues. Bassiouni *et al.,* (2011) conducted experiment to study the effect of fibrolytic enzymes supplementation on *In Situ* nutrient degradability of different complete rations and reported that percentages of *in-situ* DM, CP and CF disappearance for rations contained 60% concentrate: 40% roughage was higher than complete rations contained 40% concentrate: 60%roughage for different feedstuffs ($P<0.05$). However, Venkateswarlu *et al.,* (2014) reported inclusion of sorghum straw at 50-60% in the complete diets of Nellore lambs is considered to be economical in growing lamb's ration. In a recent study, Sakthivel *et al.,* (2016) reported that Maku lotus, a temperate legume can be fed upto 30% of dry matter intake in Sandyno weaner lambs without effecting intake and digestibility of nutrients. Sinha *et al.,* (2016) also reported that under higher plane of nutrition (TMR), there is better nutrient digestibility and energy utilization with lesser methane emission in ruminants.

References

1. Afzal, Y., Ganai, A.M., Matto, F.A. and Shad, F.I. 2009. Comparative dietaryevaluation of oats straw and tree leaves based complete feed in block and mash form in sheep. *Indian Journal of Small Ruminants* **15**(2): 212-216.

2. Bassiouni, M.I., Gaafar, H.M.A., Mohi, A.A.A., El-Din, Metwally, A.M. and Elshora, M.A.H. 2011. Evaluation of rations supplemented with fibrolytic enzyme on dairy cows performance 2. *In situ* ruminal degradability of rations containing different roughages at two concentrate to roughage ratios. *Researcher* **3**: 21-33.

3. Bhatia, T. 2004. Comparative evaluation of conventional and complete feed (mash) feeding system in sheep. *M.V.Sc., Thesis submitted to Rajasthan Agricultural University, Bikaner.*

4. Chaturvedi, O.H., Sushil, K., Mishra, A.K., Arora, A.L. and Karim, S.A. 2009. Effect of complete feed or grazing and supplementation of lambs on performance, nutrient utilization and feed cost of production. *Indian Journal of Animal Science* **79(9):** 917-920.

5. Dhuria, R.K. and Sharma, T. 2010. Nutrient utilization of bajra straw based complete feed in Magra lambs. *Indian Veterinary Journal* **87**: 1115-1117.

6. Dhuria, R.K., Sharma, T. and Garg, D.D. 2011. Mustard straw based complete feed blocks for lambs. *Indian Veterinary Journal* **11**(1): 47-49.

7. Ganai, A.M., Singh, P.K. and Ahmad, H.A. 2007. Importance of complete feed blocks in livestock production. *Livestock Line* **1**: 4.

8. Kirubanath, K., Reddy, D.N. and Naglakashmi, D. 2003. Effect of processing cotton straw based complete diet with expander-extruder on performance of crossbred calves. *Asian Australasian Journal of Animal Sciences* **16**: 11.

9. Kishore, K.R., Kumar D.S. and Ramana, J.V. 2013. Effect of feeding crop residue based complete rations on nutrient utilization in buffalo bulls. *International Journal of Agricultural Sciences and Veterinary Medicine* **1**(4): 33-42.

10. Kishore, K.R., Ramana, J.V., Kumar, D.S., Ravi, A. and Rao, E.R. 2014. Effect of feeding crop residue-based complete rations on nutrient utilization in Nellore rams. *International Journal of Small Ruminants* **20**(1): 37-40.

11. Kumar, N.N., Reddy, Y.R., Blummel, M., Nagalakshmi, D., Monika, T., Reddy, D.V.S. and Kumar, A.A. 2014. Effect of feeding differently processed sweet sorghum (*Sorghum bicolor* L. Moench) bagasse based complete diet on nutrient utilization and microbial N supply in growing ram lambs. *Small ruminant research* **1**: 52-57.

12. Lailer, P.C., Dahiya, S.S. and Chauhan, T.R. 2005. Complete feed for livestock concept, present status and future trend: A review. *Indian Journal of Animal Science* **75(1):** 84-91.

13. Malisetty, V., Yerradoddi, R.R. and Marrivada, S.R. 2013. Effect of feeding crop residues based complete rations on growth in ram lambs. *International Journal of Science, Environment and Technology* **1(2):** 15-19.

14. Mishra, A.S., Tripathi, M.K., Vaithiyanathan, S. and Jakhmola, R.C. 2013. Nutritional evaluation of fallen tree leaves as source of roughage in complete feed blocks for sheep. *Animal Nutriion and Feed Technology* **13**: 223-234.

15. Nagalakshmi, D. and Reddy, D.N. 2012. Effect of Feeding Processed Paddy Straw Based Complete Diets on Nutrient Utilization and Rumen Fermentation Pattern in Sheep. *Indian Journal of Animal Nutrition* **2**: 132-137.

16. Prasad, J. 2000. Goat, sheep and pig production and management. Kalayani Publisher, New Delhi, pp. 157.

17. Ramchandra, K. S. and Samra, J. S. 2009. Current status on data information on feed resources in different agro climatic zones in relation to nutrient requirement and availability. **In** : *Proc. of XII Animal Nutrition Conference,* January 7-9, 2006 Anand, Gujarat. pp. 1-7.

18. Reddy, G.V.N. and Reddy, M.R. (1998). Utilization of expender-extruder processed complete diet containing sunflower heads in Ongole bull calves. *Indian J. Anim. Nutr.* **15(4):** 272-275.

19. Reddy, G.V.N., Reddy, K.J. and Nagalakshmi, D. (2002). Effect of expander extruder processed complete diet containing sugarcane baggase on growth and nutrient utilization in Ongole bulls calves. *Indian J. Anim. Sci.,* **72(5):** 406-409.

20. Saini, N. and Patel, A.K. 2016. Growth performance of Magra lambs under supplementary feeding of feed block in field condition. *Proc. of XVI Biennial Animal Nutrition Conference on Innovative Approaches for Animal Feeding and Nutrition Research,* February 6-8, 2016 NDRI, Karnal, pp. 143.

21. Sakthivel, P.C., Lyue, M., Prema, N., Prabhu, M. and Sakthivadivu, R. 2016. Effect of feeding maku lotus, a temperate perennial legume, on intake and digestibility of nutrients in sandyno weaner lambs. **In** : *Proc. of XVI Biennial Animal Nutrition Conference on Innovative Approaches for Animal Feeding and Nutrition Research,* February 6-8, 2016 NDRI, Karnal, pp. 11.

22. Singh, N.P. and Sankhyan, S.K. 2003. Effect of supplementary concentrate on growth, wool yield and quality in fine wool sheep. *Animal Nutriion and Feed Technology* **3**: 189-193.

23. Sinha, S.K., Chaturvedi, V.B., Verma, A.K., Patil, A.K. and Shivani, S. 2016. Effect of feeding TMR on methane emission and energy metabolism in crossbred cattle and buffaloes. **In** : *Proc. of XVI Biennial Animal Nutrition Conference on Innovative Approaches for Animal Feeding and Nutrition Research,* February 6-8, 2016 NDRI, Karnal, pp. 94.

24. Venkateswarlu, M, Reddy, Y.R. Nagalakshmi, D. and Mahender, M. 2014. Effect of feeding sorghum straw based complete rations with different roughage to concentrate ratio on growth and carcass characteristics in Nellore ram Lambs. *Animal Nutriion and Feed Technology* **14(3):** 563.

25. Verma, D.N., Singh, S.P., Srivastava, D.K., Verma, R.B. and Prakash, OM. (2001). Performance of kids as influenced by dietary subabul. *Indian J. Anim. Nutr.,* **18(1):** 84-89.

26. Waje, S.H., Singh, S.K. and Mudgal, V. 2010. Effect of using forest grass based complete rations on growth and nutrient utilization in growing crossbred calves. *Animal Nutriion and Feed Technology* **10**: 229-234.

□□□

11

Probiotics for Better Rumen Performance in Small Ruminants

G.G. Sheikh*, A.M. Ganai, Tabinda Sehar, Vikas Mahajan and Ishfaq Ahmad

* Division of Animal Nutrition, Faculty of Veterinary Sciences and Animal Husbandry, Sher-e-Kashmir University of Agricultural Sciences and Technology of Kashmir Shuhama, Alusteng, Srinagar-190 006, Jammu and Kashmir

Many definitions have been proposed for the term "probiotic". The more widely accepted one is "live micro-organisms which, when administered in adequate amounts, confer a health benet on the host (FAO/WHO, 2002). In recent years, with increased consumer's concern about safety, quality of animal products and also environmental issues, the current purpose of using these "natural" additives is not only to increase productivity, but also to diminish the risk of animal digestive transfer of potential human pathogens, to decrease the antibiotic load and the risk of antibiotic resistance genes transfer, and to limit excretion of pollutants. The advantages of the use of probiotics in livestock are many fold like, the period of adaptation of animal is not necessary, does not hinder the management on the farm because it can be supplement to ration or mineral salt, and as probiotic is the natural product does not possess residual effect. According to Ferreira (2003), the probiotics micro-organisms most used belong to the group of lactic acid bacteria as *Lactobacillus acidophilus* and Active dry yeast products (ADYs) are generally characterized by a high concentration of viable cells (>10billion cfu/g), with the most common species being *Saccharomyces cerevisiae*. These micro-organisms are also part of the residual microbial system of the intestinal microbiota of humans and animals and these micro-organisms might rarely be involved in human and diseases (Vesterlund *et al.*, 2007). As per the reports of Guo *et al.*, (2009) *Lactobacillus acidophilus* is most tolerant to gastro-intestinal juices with highest survival rate.

1. Effect of probiotics on rumen fermentation characteristics and rumen microflora

For the efficient utilization of feed, it is important that the rumen functioning should be optimum, therefore supplementation of feed additives as well as feed technology is acceptable for livestock feeding, only when the animal maintain normal metabolism. Likewise, it is the rumen, where supplementation of probiotic brings changes in microbial ecosystem manipulating rumen fermentation to improve productivity by increasing flow of nutrients to lower part of gut. Thus, effect on rumen functioning should be thoroughly understood before bringing it to the practice. Hence, a number of scientists have conducted studies in this direction.

At birth, the rumen of the newborn is germ free, but it is very rapidly colonised by a complex and abundant microbial population. Indeed, establishment of a complex microbial ecosystem is of great importance for subsequent development of rumen function (e.g., absorption ability and feed digestion efficiency) as well as development of the immune system and for whole gut health (Hooper *et al.*, 2001). In gnotoxenic and conventional lambs fed live *S. cerevisiae* cells daily, the rate of establishment of cellulolytic bacterial population was increased and this population was more stable than in non-supplemented lambs (Chaucheyras-Durand and Fonty, 2001). Ciliate protozoa, which are not able to establish unless bacterial communities have previously colonised the rumen, appeared more rapidly in the rumen of conventional lambs in the presence of probiotics (Chaucheyras-Durand and Fonty, 2002). This supports the hypothesis that probiotics containing live yeast supplementation accelerates maturation of the rumen microbial ecosystem. This is a good example of aprobiotcs product, through its effect on early establishment of microbial communities in the rumen, having a positive impact on animal performance and health.

2. Effect of probiotics on ruminal pH and lactate accumulation

Several animal studies have reported effects of live yeasts on rumen pH stabilization. In rumen cannulated sheep receiving probiotics during their adaptation to a high concentrate diet, it has been reported that rumen pH was maintained at values compatible with an efficient rumen function, as shown by higher brolytic activities in the rumen of the supplemented animals versus controls

(Chaucheyras-Durand and Fonty, 2006). Other researchers suggested that supplementation of probiotics causes an elevation of ruminal pH (Dutta *et al.*, 2001; Kamra *et al.*, 2002; Elseed and Abusamra, 2007; Garg *et al.*, 2009; Thrune *et al.*, 2007). In these studies, higher rumen pH occurred together with lesser lactate concentrations in the rumen of supplemented animals. Stabilization of ruminal pH in the presence of probiotics has also been reported by several other authors (Bach *et al.*, 2007 and Thrune *et al.*, 2007). More than an increase in mean rumen pH, reductions in duration within a day under a certain pH threshold, as well as in area under the pH curve have been measured in the presence of live yeast probiotics (Bach *et al.*, 2007 and Thrune *et al.*, 2007).

A decrease in lactate concentration has also been reported from *in vitro* incubations with mixed ruminal micro-organisms (Lila *et al.*, 2004), which could be due to interactions between yeast cells and lactate metabolizing bacteria. Indeed, it has been shown in-vitro that one strain of *S. cerevisiae* was able to outnumber *S. bovis,* when competing for the utilization of sugars, which consequently limited the amount of lactate produced by this bacterial species (Chaucheyras *et al.*, 1996). Moreover, stimulation of growth and metabolism of lactate utilising bacteria, such as *Megasphaera elsdenii* or *Selenomonas ruminantium,* has been observed in *in-vitro* in the presence of various live yeasts (Nisbet and Martin, 1991; Rossi *et al.*, 1995; Chaucheyras *et al.*, 1996; Newbold *et al.*, 1998 and Rossi *et al.*, 2004) through a supply of growth factors, such as amino acids, peptides, vitamins and organic acids, which seemed to be essential components for lactate fermenting bacteria. These results demonstrate the potential of live yeasts to control the pH decline and so limit lactate accumulation in the rumen. However, under most practical circumstances, lactate is accumulated in the rumen only at low levels (Goad *et al.*,1998) and the fermentation pattern and decreased rumen pH are driven by high total VFA concentrations (>150mM; Brossard *et al.*, 2004). Brossard *et al.* (2006) reported effects of one strain of *S. cerevisiae* on rumen fermentations in rumen cannulated sheep fed a 600g/kg wheat grain diet, wherein live yeast was efficient at stabilising ruminal pH by stimulating ciliate Entodiniomorphid protozoa, which are known to rapidly engulf starch granules and compete effectively with amylolytic bacteria for substrate (Mendoza *et al.*, 1993; Williams and Coleman, 1997). In addition, starch is fermented by protozoa at a slower rate than by amylolytic bacteria, and the main end products of fermentation are VFA rather than lactate, which is why ciliates have a stabilizing effect in the rumen by delaying fermentation (Williams and Coleman, 1997). Moreover, Entodiniomorphs are also able to take up some of the lactate and thus, may prevent its accumulation in the rumen. Furthermore, Krizova *et al.*, (2011) and Kowalik *et al.*, (2012) also reported much higher rumen pH in animals fed probiotics supplemented ration than in the control group. The elevated rumen pH appears to be the result of the increase in number of total and cellulolytic bacteria in rumen fluid. As the bacterial population increases, requirements for rumen available nitrogen also increase and, provided that sufficient available nitrogen is present in the medium, it is logical to expect that an increased proportion of available carbon skeletons is diverted towards microbial protein synthesis rather than being fermented and producing VFA as end-products. Therefore, an increase in viable microbial cell numbers in the rumen promoted by live yeast supplementation may minimize the increase in ruminal concentrations of VFA thereby avoiding a decrease in ruminal pH.

Regarding bacterial probiotics, lactate producing bacteria (Lactobacillus), which would sustain a constant level of lactic acid, thus allowing the lactate utilising species to flourish (Nocek *et al.*, 2002; Nocek and Kautz, 2006) may represent a possible means to limit acidosis in high concentrate fed animals. Some researchers have observed either no effect or reduction in pH on yeast supplementation (El-Ghani, 2004; Brossard *et al.*, 2006; Kawas *et al.*, 2007b; Bhima *et al.*, 2009a). These variations in data between studies may be attributed to different experimental conditions related to animal (species and physiological stage), diet (composition and mode of distribution) and probiotics (strain, dose and viability).

3. Effect of probiotics on nitrogen metabolism

Because of the increasing concern of the role of livestock on climate change, nutritional strategies that aim at decreasing nitrogen loss in the rumen are of interest. Conversion of peptides and amino acids to ammonia in the rumen is unfavourable to the host animal, as energy is required for microbial protein synthesis, and not all ammonia is incorporated into protein (Wallace *et al.*, 1997a). Data reporting effects of probiotics on nitrogen microbial metabolism in the rumen are scarce and somewhat controversial as the parameter considered while assessing the impact of yeasts *in-vivo* is ammonia concentration depend on nature of the diet, host and rumen microbial related factors.

However, as per Chaucheyras-Durand and Fonty, (2001) in genotobiotically reared lambs, ammonia concentration decreased in the presence of a probiotics a phenomenon also observed in the rumen of newborn lambs (Chaucheyras-Durand and Fonty, 2002). The reduced level of ammonia nitrogen on feed additives supplementation may not be associated with increase the digestion of DM and NDF, more energy substrates are released, improving microbial protein synthesis by reducing the concentration of N-NH_3 (Gado *et al.*, 2011) and increased uptake and assimilation of ammonia nitrogen by rumen microbes due to stimulation of bacterial growth. The results corroborate well with the reports where reduced ammonia nitrogen concentration were found in rumen due to probiotic supplementation (Singla *et al.*, 2000; Kamra *et al.*, 2002; El-Ghani *et al.*, 2004; Bhima *et al.*, 2009a; Garg *et al.*, 2009; Malik and Singh, 2009; Hillal *et al.*, 2011; Comert *et al.*, 2015; Ganai *et al.*, 2015; Shankhpal *et al.*, 2016). However, several reports (Kawas *et al.*, 2007b; Brossard *et al.*, 2006; Elseed and Abusamra *et al.*, 2007; Thrune *et al.*, 2009) indicated either no change or numerical increase in NH_3-N on yeast supplementation. Dietary inclusion of probiotic culture had a small influence on rumen fermentation parameters and *in-vivo* digestibility but its effect on nitrogen metabolism appears to be dependent on nitrogen content of the basal diets (Moloney and Drennan, 1994). However, Shankhpal *et al.*, (2016), Kumar and Dutta *et al.* (2016) and Bhima *et al.*, (2009a) reported that supplementing yeast to kids significantly improved total N and lowered NH_3-N with no effect on TCA precipitated nitrogen. *In-vitro* ndings indicated that one yeast strain could inuence growth and activity of proteolytic rumen bacteria, by limiting their action on protein and peptides. The mechanisms of yeast action may be due to competition between live *S. cerevisiae* cells and bacteria for energy supply and by a direct inhibitory effect of yeasts' small peptides on bacterial peptidases (Chaucheyras-Durand *et al.*, 2005). Combined, these data suggest some changes in the N metabolism of rumen micro-organisms in the presence of probiotics.

4. Effect of probiotics on hydrogen metabolism and methane mitigation

Methanogenesis is an essential metabolic pathway for hydrogen elimination and subsequently for efficient degradation of plant cell wall carbohydrates in the rumen (Ushida and Jouany, 1996; Wolin *et al.*, 1997). Relative to probiotics, there is little information dealing with their potential effects on hydrogen transfer mechanisms and methanogenesis. One mechanism of action could be to shift H_2 utilization from methanogenesis to reductive acetogenesis. *In-vitro* studies have shown beneficial effects of feeding a live yeast strain on growth and H_2-utilisation and acetate production by acetogenic bacteria isolated from a rumen of lambs, even in the presence of methanogens (Chaucheyras *et al.*, 1995a; Chaucheyras-Durand *et al.*, 1997), but these effects have not been veried *in vivo*. Similarly, methane production of beef cattle, expressed as a proportion of gross energy intake, was not impacted by the presence of yeast strain (McGinn *et al.*, 2004). Lynch and Martin (2002) reported a 20% decrease in methane production after a 48h of incubation of mixed rumen micro-organisms in the presence of alfalfa and a live yeast product.

Studies with other yeast strains have been conflicting, reporting either no effect in stulated sheep (Mathieu *et al.*, 1996), and *in vitro* (Lila *et al.*, 2004), or an increase in methane production in batch cultures with mixed rumen microora (Martin *et al.*, 1989). Evaluation of various yeast strains in rumen-simulating fermenters on methane production reported a strong strain effect, with results ranging from no effect in one study to a 58% decrease in another (Newbold and Rode, 2006). In a recent study, Priambodo *et al.* (2009) reported also reported similar findings that probiotics supplementation has no effect on methane production. Future work will be then necessary to further investigate the role of probiotics sasecological tools to control methane emissions from the rumen.

5. Effect of probiotics on microbial communities

The main factors implicated in the beneficial effect of probiotics on rumen micro-organisms is due to the capacity of yeast cells to scavenge ruminal oxygen. Studies have also reported that redox potential of rumen fluid was lowered in the presence of live yeasts in lambs (Chaucheyras-Durand *et al.*, 2002), in sheep (Mathieu *et al.*, 1996) suggesting that live yeast cells could create more favourable environmental conditions for growth and activities of the rumen microbiota. Bhanderi *et al.* (2016) reported total anaerobic and total cellulolytic bacteria concentration was significantly ($P<0.05$) higher in yeast supplemented groups. Lascano *et al.* (2009) found yeast addition increased number of viable bacteria cells in ruminants with bacterial counts decreased for the first 2 h after feeding then increased 4 h post feeding. Saro *et al.* (2012) reported that total bacterial DNA concentrations decreased at 4 h after feeding and then increased at 8 h after feeding to values similar ($P > 0.05$) to those before feeding. Similar results have been reported for sheep (Martin and Michalet-Doreau, 1995; Michalet-Doreau *et al.*, 2002). In young pre-ruminants, bacterial probiotics, such as lactic acid bacteria (Lactobacillus spp.) generally target the small intestine, as the rumen is not yet developed, and they represent an interesting means to stabilise the gut microbiota and limit the risk of pathogen colonisation. The effectiveness of some yeast strains to stimulate growth or/and activities of fibrolytic bacteria has also been demonstrated. *In-vitro*, a *S. cerevisiae* strain stimulated growth of *Fibrobacter succinogenes S85* and reduced the lag time for growth of *Ruminococcus albus 7, Ruminococcus flavefaciens FD1* and *Butyrivibrio fibrisolvens D1* (Girard *et al.*, 1995). Callaway and Martin *et al.* (1997) showed that the same yeast could accelerate the rate, but not the extent, of cellulose filter paper degradation by *F. succinogenesS85* and *R. flavefaciens FD1*. *In-vivo*, in gnotoxenic lambs harbouring three species of bacteria (*F. succinogenes, R. albus* and *R. flavefaciens*) as sole cellulolytic organisms, cellulolytic bacteria became established earlier and remained at a high and stable level even after a stressful period (lambs were fitted with a rumen cannula) in the lambs receiving a probiotic yeast daily (Chaucheyras-Durand *et al.*, 2001). Fibre degradation processes would thereby be set up more efficiently in the early age of the animal, as shown by the increase in polysaccharidase and glycoside-hydrolase activities in the presence of yeast in the rumen of genotoxenic lambs (Chaucheyras-Durand *et al.*, 2001). The proportions of 16S rRNA of *F. succinogenes, R. albus* and *R. flavefaciens* have been shown to increase in the rumen of sheep receiving another yeast product (Chaucheyras *et al.*, 1997). A 2 to 4 fold increase in the number of 16S rRNA gene copies of *R. albus* and *R. flavefaciens* was also measured with real-time PCR in rumen contents of sheep receiving a high-concentrate diet and a live yeast probiotic (Mosoni *et al.*, 2007). Chaucheyras-Durand *et al.* (2010) reported that the supplementation of 10^{10} cfu/day/cow of the yeast additive promoted colonization of fibrous substrates by cellulolytic bacteria (*F. succinogenes, R. flavefaciens, B. fibrisolvens*) and fungi but that the degree of stimulation was depending on the nature of the substrate, and on the microbial species targeted. It was noticed that feedstuffs with highest levels of lignin and thereby with less easily accessible digestible carbohydrates were better degraded in the presence of yeast, suggesting a particularly marked impact on the microbial breakdown of lignin polysaccharide linkeages.

Ruminal fungi are considered to be primary colonizers of plant biomass (Edwards *et al.*, 2008). Saro *et al.* (2012) reported relative abundance of fungal DNA values at 4 h after feeding on solid rumen contents, compared with those at 0 and 8 h for both diets, which is in agreement with the less relative abundance of fungal DNA observed in our study at 2 h after feeding in rumen fluid. The possible reason for positive effect of probiotics supplementation on fungal count may be supply of thiamine, a vitamin required by rumen fungi for zoosporogenesis (Chaucheyras-Durand *et al.*, 2010). Similar results were reported by (Chaucheyras *et al.*, 1995), found fungal zoospore germination and cellulose degradation were increased in the presence of a strain of *S. cerevisiae.* The authors suggested that yeasts could enhance fungal colonization of plant cell walls, which was confirmed recently (Chaucheyras-Durand *et al.*, 2010). In the same studies, cellulose lter paper degradation by *N. frontalis* was also stimulated in the presence of live yeast cells. A stimulatory effect of a heat labile and proteinase *A. oryzae* extract on growth and cellulase production by pure cultures of *Neocallimastix, Orpinomyces* and *Piromyces* has been reported in other studies (Welch *et al.*, 1996).

The mechanism which could be implicated in the interaction between probiotics and protozoa are not currently known. Probiotics may provide nutrients to the protozoal cells, or enhanced anaerobic conditions by oxygen scavenging as already described by (Chaucheyras and Fonty, 2002). The other probable reason may be the pH of the rumen liquor. Generally, slightly alkaline ruminal pH favours ruminal protozoa growth, while their growth is disturbed when pH falls below 6.0 and rumen protozoa are completely eliminated at pH 5.5 and below (Hungate, 1966).

Ciliate protozoa, which are not able to establish unless bacterial communities have previously colonized the rumen (Fonty *et al.*, 1988), appeared more rapidly in the rumen of conventional lambs in the presence of live yeasts (Chaucheyras-Durand *et al.*, 2002).This supports the hypothesis that live yeast supplementation accelerates maturation of the rumen microbial ecosystem. Kowalik *et al.* (2012), Brossard *et al.* (2006) and Arakaki *et al.* (2000) also reported the supplementation with metabolites of yeast led to numerically higher ciliate numbers. Ganai (2011) reported that total protozoal counts in different treatment groups suggested that supplementation of yeast alone and in combination with enzyme as well as time of sampling had highly significant effect on total protozoal count. Although the effects of yeast and protozoa are still imperfectly known, several studies have reported numerical increase in rumen protozoal population (Garcia *et al.*, 2000; Singla *et al.*, 2000; Brossard *et al.*, 2006; Garg *et al.*, 2009) due to yeast supplementation.

Conclusion

Probiotics may improve growth, feed intake, digestibility, ruminal microflora and increase the ruminal fermentation with improvement in rumen pH. So, their effect on the fiber digestion may be more intense in small ruminants receiving high concentrate diets. It is further stated that inclusion of probiotics in the diet will improve the physiological health status of animals.

References

1. Arakaki, L.C., Stahringer, R.C., Garrett, J.E., Dehority, B.A. 2000. The effects of feeding monensin and yeast culture, alone or in combination, on the concentration and generic composition of rumen protozoa in steers fed on low-quality pasture supplemented with increasing levels of concentrate. Animal Feed Science and Technology **84:** 121-127.

2. Bach, A., Iglesias, C. and Devant, M. 2007. Daily rumen pH pattern of loose housed dairy cattle as affected by feeding pattern and live yeast supplementation. Animal Feed Science and Technology **136:** 156-163.

3. Bhanderi, B.M., Parnekar, S., Shankhpal, S. and Thube, H. 2016. Effect of supplementing live yeast culture on rumen fermentation, nutrient digestibility and biochemical profile in kankrej cows.*Proc. of XVI Biennial Animal Nutrition Conference on Innovative Approaches for Animal Feeding and Nutrition Research,* February 6-8, 2016 NDRI, Karnal. pp.15.

4. Bhima, B., Reddy, Y.R., Pavani, M., Reddy, M. S. and Rao. L.V. 2009a. Rumen fermentation pattern in Murrah buffalo steers fed on straw based complete diet supplemented with thermotolerant probiotic yeast (Saccharomyces cerevisiae) at graded levels. Indian Journal of Animal Nutrition **26(3):** 239-342.

5. Brossard, L., Chaucheyras-Durand, F., Michalet-Doreau, B. and Martin, C. 2006. Dose effect of live yeasts on rumen microbial communities and fermentations during butyric latent acidosis in sheep: new type of interaction. *Anim. Sci.* **82:** 829-836.

6. Brossard, L., Martin, C., Chaucheyras-Durand, F., Michalet Doreau, B., 2004. Protozoa involved in butyric rather than lactic fermentative pattern during latent acidosis in sheep. *Reprod. Nutr. Dev.* **44:** 195-206.

7. Callaway, E.S. and Martin, S.A. 1997. Effects of *Saccharomyces cerevisiae* culture on ruminal bacteira that utilize lactate and digest cellulose. *Journal of Dairy Science* **50**: 2035-2044.

8. Chaucheyras, D.F. and Fonty, G. 2002. Rumen microbial ecology and *Saccharomyces cerevisiae* CNCM 1-1077. Journal of Dairy Science **85 (Suppl. 1):** 356.

9. Chaucheyras, D.F., Fonty, G., Bertin, G. and Gouet, P. 1995. Effect of live *Saccharomyces cerevisiae* cells on zoospore germination, growth and cellulolytic activity of of the rumen anaerobic fungus. *Neocallimastix frontalis* MCH 3. *Curr. Microbiol.* **3:** 201-205.

10. Chaucheyras, F., Fonty, G., Bertin, G., Gouet, P., 1995a. In-vitro H2 utilization by a ruminal acetogenic bacterium cultivated alone or in association with an archaea methanogen is stimulated by a probiotic strain of *Saccharomyces cerevisiae. Appl. Environ. Microbiol.* **61:** 3466-3467.

11. Chaucheyras, F., Fonty, G., Bertin, G., Gouet, P., 1995b. Effects of live *Saccharomyces cerevisiae* cells on zoospore germination, growth, and cellulolytic activity of the rumen anaerobic fungus, *Neocallimastix frontalis MCH3.Curr.Microbiol.* **31:** 201-205.

12. Chaucheyras, F., Fonty, G., Bertin, G., Salmon, J.M., Gouet, P. 1996. Effects of a strain of *Saccharomyces cerevisiae* (LevucellSC), a microbial additive for ruminants, on lactate metabolism *in-vitro. Can. J. Microbiol.* **42:** 927-933.

13. Chaucheyras-Durand, F. and Fonty, G. 2001. Establishment of cellulolytic bacteria and development of fermentative activities in the rumen of gnotobiotically-reared lambs receiving the microbial additive Saccharomyces cerevisiae CNCM I-1077.*Reprod. Nutr. Dev.* **41:** 57-68.

14. Chaucheyras Durand, F. and Fonty, G. 2002. Inuence of a probiotic yeast (*Saccharomyces cerevisiae CNCMI-1077*) on microbial colonization and fermentation in the rumen of newborn lambs. *Microb. Ecol. Health Dis.* **14:** 30-36.

15. Chaucheyras Durand, F. and Fonty, G. 2006.Effects and modes of action of live yeasts in the rumen.*Biologia (Bratislava)* **61(6):** 741-750.

16. Chaucheyras-Durand, F., Ameilbonne, A., Walker, N.D., Mosoni, P. and Forano, E. 2010. Effect of a live yeast, *Saccharomyces cerevisiae I-1077* on in situ ruminal degradation of alfalfa hay and fibre-associated micro-organisms. *J. Anim. Sci.* **88(E-Suppl. 2)** 145.

17. Chaucheyras-Durand, F., Fonty, G. and Bertin, G. 1997.Effects of a microbial additive, Levucell SC, on growth and metabolism of a ruminal acetogenic bacterial strain in-vitro. In: Proceedings of Rumen Function Conference, Chicago, USA, p. 33.

18. Cömert, M., [a]ayan, Y., Ozelçam, H and G.Y. Baykal. 2015. Effects of *Saccharomyces cerevisiae* supplementation and anhydrous ammonia treatment of wheat straw on in-situ degradability and, rumen fermentation and growth performance of yearling lambs. *Asian Australas. J. Anim. Sci.* **5:** 639-646.

19. Dutta, T.K., Kundu, S.S. and Sharma, D.D. 2001. Potential of probiotics supplementation on *in-vitro* rumen fermentation and ^{35}S incorporation in microbial protein. Indian Journal of Animal Nutrition **18(3):** 227-234.

20. Edwards, J.E., Kingston-Smith, A.H., Jimenez, H. R., Huws, S. A., Skøt, K. P., Grifth, G.W., McEwan, N. R. and Theodorou. M.K. 2008. Dynamics of initial colonization of non-conserved perennial ryegrass by anaerobic fungi in the bovine rumen. *FEMS Microbiol. Ecol.* **66:** 537–545.

21. El-Ghani, A.A. 2004. Influence of diet supplementation with yeast culture (*Saccharomyces cerevisiae*) on performance of Zaraibi goats. *Small Rumin.Res.* pp. 223-229.

22. Elseed, F.A.M.A., Rania, Abusamra, M.A. 2007. Effect of supplemental yeast (*Saccharomyces cerevisiae*) culture on NDF digestibility and rumen fermentation of forage sorghum hay in Nubian goats kids. *Res. J. Biol. Sci.* **3(3):** 133-137.

23. FAO/WHO. 2002. Report of a joint FAO/WHO expert consultation on guidelines for the evaluation of probiotics in food. London, Ontario, Canada: World Health Organization and Food Agriculture Organization of the United Nations.

24. Ferreira C.L.L.F. 2003. Grupo de aplicacao technologica de bacterias probioticas In: prebioticos e probioticos: Atualizacaoe prospeccdo, pp 07-33 viscosa, Brasil: UFV.

25. Fonty, G., Senaud, J., Jouany, J.P. and Gouet, P. 1988. Establishment of ciliate protozoa in the rumen of conventional and conventionalized lambs: inuence of diet and management conditions. *Can. J. Microbiol.* **34:** 235-241.

26. Gado H.M., Salem, A.Z.M., Odongo, N.E. and Borhami, B.E. 2011. Influence of exogenous enzymes ensiled with orange pulp on digestion and growth performance in lambs. *Anim Nutr. Feed Technol.* **165:** 131-136.

27. Ganai, A.M., Sharma, T. and Dhuria, R.K. 2011. Influence of exogenous fibrolytic enzymes on in-vitro fermentation of bajra straw in goats. Veteri.Pract. **12:** 2.

28. Ganai, A.M., Sharma, T. and Dhuria, R.K. 2015. Effect of yeast (Saccharomyces cervevisiae) supplementation on ruminal digestion of bajra (Pennisetum glaucum) straw and bajra starw based complete feed in-vitro. Anim. Nutri. Feed tech. **15:** 145-153.

29. Garcia, C.C.G., Mendoza, M. G.D., Gonzalez, M.S., Cobos, P.M., Ortega, C.M. E. and Ramirez, L.R. 2000. Effect of yeast culture (*Saccharomyces cerevisiae*) and monensin on ruminal fermentation and digestion in sheep. Animal Feed Science and Technology **83:** 165-170.

30. Garg, D.D., Sharma, T. and Dhuria R.K. 2009. Effect of groundnut straw based complete feed alone and in combination with yeast in ration of sheep. *Anim. Nutr. Feed Tech.* **9:** 137-144.

31. Girard, I.D. and Dawson K.A. 1995. Effect of a yeast culture on growth characteristics of representative ruminal bacteria. Journal of Animal Science **73:** 264.

32. Goad, D.W., Goad, C.L. and Nagaraja, T.G. 1998. Ruminal microbial and fermentative changes associated with experimentally induced subacute acidosis in steers. *Journal of Animal Science* **76**: 234-241.

33. Hillal, H., El-Sayaad, G. and Abdella, M. 2011. Effect of growth promoters (probiotics) supplementation on performance, rumen activity and some blood constituents in growing lambs. Archiv Tierzucht **54:** 607-617.

34. Hooper, L.V., Wong, M.H., Thelin, A., Hansson, L., Falk, P.G. and Gordon, J.I. 2001. Molecular analysis of commensal host-microbial relationships in the intestine. Science **291:** 881-884.

35. Hungate, R. E. 1966. The rumen and its microbes. Academic Press, New York.

36. Kamra, D.N., Chaudhary, L.C., Agarwal, N., Singh, R., Pathak, N.N. and Agarwal, N. 2002. Growth performance, nutrient utilization, rumen fermentation and enzyme activities in calves fed on *Saccharomyces cerevisiae* supplemented diets. Indian Journal of Animal Science **72(6):** 472-475.

37. Kawas, J.R., Garcia-Castillo, R., Fimbres-Durazo, H., Garza-Cazares, F., Hernandez-Vidal, J.F.G., Fimbres-Durazo, H., Olivares-Saenz, E. and Lu, C.D. 2007b. Effect of sodium bicarbonate and yeast on nutrient intake, digestibility and ruminal fermentation of live-weight lambs fed finishing diets. Small Ruminant Research **67:** 149-156.

38. Kowalik B., Skomia³, J., Paj¹k, J.J., Taciak, M., Majewska, M. and Be³¿ecki, G. 2012. Population of ciliates, rumen fermentation indicators and biochemical parameters of blood serum in heifers fed diets supplemented with yeast (*Saccharomyces cerevisiae*) preparation. Animal Science Papers and Reports **30:** 329-338.

39. Køížová, L., Richter, M., Tøináctý, J., Øíha, J. and Kumprechtová, D. 2011. The effect of feeding live yeast cultures on ruminal pH and redox potential in dry cows as continuously measured by a new wireless device. Czech Journal of Animal Science **56:** 37-45.

40. Kumar, M. and Dutta, T.K. 2016. Effect of yeast culture (*Saccharomyces cerevisiae*) supplementing on rumen fermentation of Pregnant Barbari goats. *Proc. of XVI Biennial Animal Nutrition Conference on Innovative Approaches for Animal Feeding and Nutrition Research,* February 6-8, 2016 NDRI, Karnal. pp. 29.

41. Lascano G.J., Zanton, G.I. and Heinrichs, A.J. 2009. Concentrate level and *Saccharomyces cerevisiae* affect rumen fluid associated bacteria numbers in dairy heifers. Livestock Science **126:** 189-194.

42. Lila, Z.A., Mohammed, N., Yasui, T., Kurokawa, Y., Kanda, S. and Itabashi, H. 2004. Effect of a twin starin of *Saccharomyces cerevisiae* live cells on mixed ruminal micro-organisms fermentation in vitro. Journal of Animal Science **82:** 1847-1854.

43. Lynch, H.A. and Martin, S.A. 2002. Effects of *Saccharomyces cerevisiae* culture and *Saccharomyces cerevisiae* live cells on *in-vitro* mixed ruminal microorganism fermentation. Journal of Dairy Science **85:** 2603-2608.

44. Malik, R. and Singh, R. 2009. Effect of yeast and fungi culture on in-vitro ruminal fermentation. Indian Journal of Animal Nutrition **26:** 40-45.

45. Martin, C. and Michalet-Doreau, B. 1995. Variations in mass and enzyme activity of rumen microorganisms: Effect of barley and buffer supplements. Journal of Food Agricultural Science **67:** 407–413.

46. Martin, S.A., Nisbet, D.J. and Dean, R.G. 1989. Influence of a commercial yeast supplement on *in-vitro* ruminal fermentation. Nutrition Reports International **40:** 395-403.

47. Mathieu, F., Jouany, Senaud, P., Bohatier, J., Bertin, J. and Mercier, M. 1996. The effect of *Saccharomyces cerevisiae* and *Aspergillus oryzae* on fermentation in the rumen of faunated and defaunated sheep. Protozoal and probiotic interactions. Reproduction Nutrition Development **36(3):** 271-287.

48. McGinn, S.M., Beauchemin, K.A., Coates, T. and Colombatto, D. 2004. Methane emissions from beef cattle: effects of monensin, sunower oil, enzymes, yeast, and fumaric acid. Journal of Animal Science **82:** 3346–3356.

49. Mendoza, G.D., Britton, R.A. and Stock, R.A. 1993. Influence of ruminal protozoa on site and extent of starch digestion and ruminal fermentation. Journal of Animal Science **71:** 1572–1578.

50. Michalet-Doreau, B., Fernandez, I. and Fonty, G. 2002. A comparisonof enzymatic and molecular approaches to characterize the cellulolytic microbial ecosystems of the rumen and the ceacum. Journal of Animal Science **80:** 790–796.

51. Moloney, A.P. and Drennan, M.J. 1994. The influence of the basal diet on the effects of yeast culture on ruminal fermentation and digestion. Animal Feed Science Technology **50:** 55-73.

52. Mosoni, P., Chaucheyras-Durand, F., Béra-Maillet, C. and Forano, E. 2007. Quantication by real-time PCR of cellulolytic bacteria in the rumen of sheep after supplementation of a forage diet with readily fermentable carbohydrates.Effect of a yeast additive. *Journal of Applied Microbiology* **103:** 2676-2685.

53. Newbold, C.J. and Rode, L.M., 2006. Dietary additives to control methanogenesis in the rumen. *Int.Congr.Ser.* **1293:** 138-147.

54. Newbold, C.J., McIntosh, F.M. and Wallace, R.J. 1998. Changes in the microbial population of a rumen-simulating fermenter in response to yeast culture.*Can.* Journal of Animal Science **78:** 241-244.

55. Nisbet, D.J. and Martin, S.A. 1991.Effects of *Saccharomyces cerevisiae* culture on lactate utilization by the ruminal bacterium *Selenomonas ruminantium*. Journal of Animal Science **69:** 4628–4633.

56. Nocek, J.E. 1997. Bovine acidosis: implications on laminitis. *Journal of Dairy Science* **80**: 1005-1028.

57. Nocek, J.E. and Kautz, W.P. 2006. Direct-fed microbial supplementation on ruminal digestion, health, and performance of pre and postpartum dairy cattle. *Journal of Dairy Science* **89**: 260-266.

58. Priambodo, T.W., Hummel, J., Kehraus, S. and Südekum, K.H. 2009. *In vitro* evaluation of four bacterial species as potential probiotics in

the rumen.University of Bonn, Bonn, Germany. Journal of Animal Science 87, E-Suppl.

59. Rossi, F., Luccia, A.D., Vincenti, D. and Cocconcelli, P.S. 2004. Effects of peptidic fractions from Saccharomyces cerevisiae culture on growth and metabolism of the ruminal bacteria *Megasphaera elsdenii*. Animal Research **53:** 177-186.

60. Rossi, F.P.S., Cocconcelli and Masoero, F. 1995. Effect of a *Saccharomyces cerevisiae* culture on growth and lactate utilization by the ruminal bacterium *Megasphaera elsdenii*. Annual Zootechnica **44:** 403.

61. Saro, C., Ranilla, M.J. and Carro, M.D. 2012.Postprandial changes of fiber-degrading microbes in the rumen of sheep fed diets varying in type of forage as monitored by real-time PCR and automated ribosomal intergenic spacer analysis. Journal of Animal Science **90:** 4487-4494.

62. Shankhpal, S., Patel, G.R., Subash Parnekar, Agarwal, A., Kumar, D. and Pathan, S. 2016. Effect of bypass fat feeding bypass fat and yeast (*Saccharomyces cerevisiae*) supplemented total mixed ration in weaner Surti kids. *Proc. of XVI Biennial Animal Nutrition Conference on Innovative Approaches for Animal Feeding and Nutrition Research,* February 6-8, 2016 NDRI, Karnal. pp. 300.

63. Singla, M., Kumar, U., Sareen, K.V. Singh, S. 2000. Effect of yeast culture (YEA-SACC1026) supplement on fermentation and in *sacco* digestibility of some roughages in buffalo calves. Indian Journal of Animal Science **70(3):** 289-293.

64. Thrune, M., Bach, A., Ruiz-Moreno, M., Stern, M.D., Linn, J.G. 2007. Effects of *Saccharomyces cerevisiae* on ruminal pH and microbial fermentation in lactating dairy cows. Journal of Dairy Science **90(Suppl. 1)** 172.

65. Ushida, K. and Jouany, J.P. 1996. Methane production associated with rumen-ciliated protozoa and its effect on protozoan activity. *Letters in Applied Microbiology* **23:** 129-132.

66. Vesterlund, S., Vankerckhoven, V., Saxelin, M., Goossens, H., Salminen, S. and Ouwehand, A.C. 2007. Safety assessment of Lactobacillus strains: presence of putative risk factors infaecal, blood and probiotic isolates. *International Journal of Food Microbiology* **116:** 325-331

67. Wallace, R.J., Onodera, R. and Cotta, M.A., 1997a. Metabolism of nitrogen-containing compounds. In: Hobson, P.N., Stewart, C.S.

(Eds.), The Rumen Microbial Ecosystem, second ed. Chapman & Hall, London, UK, pp. 283-328.

68. Welch, R.P., Tsai, K.P.E., Harper, G., Chang, J.S. and Calza, R.E. 1996. The effect of *Aspergillus oryzae* fermentation extract on the anaerobic fungus *Neocallimastix frontalis* EB 188: Effects on physiology. *Applierd Microbiology and Biotechnol*ogy **45:** 811-816.

69. Williams, A.G. and Coleman, G.S. 1997. The rumen protozoa. In: Hobson, P.N., Stewart, C.S. (Eds.), The Rumen Microbial Ecosystem, second ed. Chapman & Hall, London, UK, pp. 73-139.

70. Wolin, M.J., Miller, T.L. and Stewart, C.S. 1997. Microbe–microbe interactions. In: Hobson, P.N., Stewart, C.S. (Eds.), The Rumen Microbial Ecosystem, second ed. Chapman & Hall, London, UK, pp. 467-491.

□□□

12

Role of Next Generation Sequencing in Wildlife Forensics

Kajal Kumar Jadav* and Vikas Mahajan

*School of Wildlife Forensic & Health, NDVSU, Jabalpur

Since the introduction of the Sanger sequencing method in the 1970s (Sanger *et al.*, 1977), DNA sequencing technology has enabled enormous advances in molecular biology and genetics. Several large projects have been successfully completed using this technology, such as the Human Genome Project, Rice Genome Project and Swine Genome Project, as well as genome projects of many other species.

Capillary Electrophosresis (CE) based assays served the forensic community well for the past two decades, they also bear limitations in throughput, scalability, and allelic resolution. For example, CE limits the total number and classes of loci that can be multiplexed together. This is due in part to the restriction on the number of loci that can be amplified and detected simultaneously to avoid size overlap of fluorescently tagged amplicons. The maximum number to date is limited to ~24 loci using CE (Wang *et al.*, Oostdik *et al.*, 2014; 2015). Second, CE-based assays don't accommodate sample multiplexing and, therefore, samples must be processed individually. Third, CE-based analysis with length-based typing cannot capture sequence differences present in alleles of the same length. This impedes mixture detection and resolution. Fourth, CE-based typing may not provide complete results on forensic DNA casework samples containing low amounts of template DNA that are either degraded, inhibited, or both. Thus, decisions may be required to determine which assay/workflow might be most effective with these limited, degraded samples *a priori*. Iterative testing utilizes more input DNA with each kit or method attempted, in search of a "full profile." Sixth, in the event of exclusionary results or no DNA database hit, CE-based STR DNA results do not provide investigative lead information, and result in a genetic dead end.

However, disadvantages of the conventional Sanger sequencing technology, including its low throughput, high cost and operation difficulties, have limited its use in deeper and more complex genome analyses (Fullwood, *et al.*, 2009). NGS technology refers to non-Sanger-based high-throughput DNA sequencing technology. Millions or billions of DNA molecules can be sequenced in parallel, thereby increasing the throughput substantially and minimizing the need for the fragment-cloning method often used in Sanger sequencing. It includes second-generation sequencing technology based on loop array sequencing, which can analyze a large number of samples simultaneously, as well as third-generation sequencing technology, which can determine the base composition of single DNA molecules.

Major advances in NGS now provide low cost, large-volume sequencing capabilities that are actively applied to various questions in areas, such as evolutionary biology (Berglund *et al.*, 2011), oncology, (Kothari *et al.*, 2014), microbial genomics (Budowle *et al.*, 2014) agrigenomics (Kawahara *et al.*, 2013) and disease genomics (Pihlstrøm *et al.*, 2014) worldwide. Next-generation sequencing, also known as massively parallel sequencing, has been around for over a decade (Van *et al.*, 2014). NGS enables to address limitations of capillary electrophoresis in forensic testing (Zascavage *et al.*, 2013; Borsting *et al.*, 2015). In addition to the ability to multiplex ~10-fold more loci than current CE-based systems, other advantages include:

- Sample-specific barcoding for multiplexing up to 96 samples per analysis using 1 ng or less of template DNA.The combination of sample and locus multiplexing can replace a minimum of 6 separate CE-based kits.
- Sequence variant detection reveals additional STR alleles of the same size that are not detected by CE (Gettings *et al.*, 2015). These "isometric heterozygotes," or isoalleles, can be visually displayed in the software (Illumina Inc, 2015). This nucleotide-based genotyping can tease out the number of contributors to aid mixture resolution. Sequence differences can distinguish an allele of a minor contributor and the stutter of a major contributor, even if they are of the same amplicon length. In CE, these data appear as one peak. In some mixtures, CE data indicate a single source sample or a two-person mixture, whereas NGS detects

three or more DNA contributors. Genetic data from mixed sample studies, with major:minor ratios from 99.9:0.1% to 50:50%, indicate the ability to detect shared and unshared (unique, obligate) minor contributor alleles at less than 5% of the major donor.

- Enhanced results on degraded and inhibited DNA samples, as the targets of the majority of the loci are <200 bp, generated in a single reaction.
- Compatibility with worldwide STR DNA databases created with CE methods, and
- Ability to investigate familial relationships and personal identification using X and Y STRs, without iterative testing. This reduces consumption of DNA samples and the need for deciding which assay to implement, as all classes of forensically significant loci are amplified in one forensic NGS multiplex. Forensic scientists over the globe are actively investigating and implementing NGS systems for forensic genomics due to their ability to improve DNA typing (Caratti *et al.*, 2015; Hussing *et al.*, 2015). By delivering targeted data on forensically significant loci, forensic scientists can answer a wider range of questions in a single assay.

In Wildlife Forensic Science congress, 2005, a scientist called Budowle and his colleagues commented on the increasing use of genetic analysis used to distinguish animal products in forensic cases. Budowle and his colleagues additionally highlighted the requirement of quality practices and pointed towards human DNA forensic analyses, as a model from which recommendations and guidelines may be discussed for wildlife forensics.

Overview of NGS technology

In 2005, Roche introduced the 454 Genome Sequencing System (Margulies *et al.*, 2005), the world's first pyrosequencing-based high-throughput sequencing system. The first 454 Genome Sequencer was capable of generating approximately 200,000 reads of 110 base pairs (bp) in length (the current maximum read length is 1000 bp). In 2007, Applied Biosystems (ABI) introduced the SOLID second-generation sequencing system based on the oligonucleotide ligation technique and two-base encoding system, whereas Illumina released Solexa sequencing technology. The Illumina and SOLID sequencers generated much larger numbers of reads than the 454 system (30 and 100 million reads, respectively); nonetheless, the reads produced were only 35 bp long. In 2010, Ion Torrent, a faster and low-cost sequencer based on semiconductor technology, was introduced. This sequencer does not rely on fluorescence, chemiluminescence, or enzyme cascades for sequencing signal detection. Currently, a maximum read length of up to 400 bp can be obtained using this system.

All these new sequencing methods have led to three major improvements from the conventional technologies. First, these technologies do not require bacterial cloning of DNA fragments; instead, they rely on the preparation of NGS libraries in a cell-free system. Second, instead of hundreds of sequencing reactions, they can parallelize the thousands-to-many-millions of sequencing reaction. Third, the sequencing output is directly detected with no need for electrophoresis. The enormous number of reads generated by NGS enabled the sequencing of entire genomes at an unprecedented speed and thus it came to be widely used in various fields of life sciences. However, one drawback of second-generation sequencing technology is its relatively short read lengths, which has resulted in difficulties in subsequent sequence splicing, assembly, annotation and bioinformatics analysis (Wang *et al.*, 2015). Furthermore, standard PCR was used to randomly amplify genomic fragments during library preparation. Due to the complex structure of genomes, factors, such as secondary structure and thermal stability will affect the efficiency of PCR amplification. Therefore, the complete genomic sequence may not be represented in the library produced by such amplification. This can be problematic due to the relative deviation between amplified and non-amplified DNA molecules, resulting in potential inaccuracies in gene expression analysis. This concern is particularly relevant for highly-expressed genes (Oostdik *et al.*, 2014). Moreover, these shortcomings have restricted the application and development of second-generation sequencing technology to some extent and have necessitated the development of third-generation single-molecule sequencing technology (Berglund *et al.*, 2011; Kothari *et al.*, 2014; Van *et al.*, 2014).

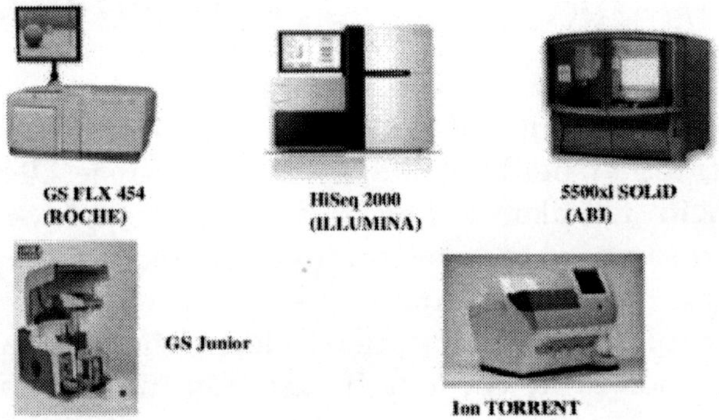

The third-generation sequencing technology not only allows the detection of single molecules but also enables real-time sequencing. The current leader in this field is the PacBio RS system (Pacific Biosciences), which utilizes the single-molecule, real-time (SMRT) DNA sequencing technology. SMRT sequencing is based on the sequencing-by-synthesis approach; an SMRT chip contains thousands of zero-mode waveguides, in which the DNA polymerase molecules used to synthesize the DNA fragments of interest are attached. Compared to second-generation sequencing, the latest SMRT technology can achieve an average read lengths of 5500"8500 bp. Moreover, it can also directly detect epigenetic modifications, such as 4-methylctosine (mC), 5-mC and 6-methyladenine (mA) (Budowle *et al.*, 2014).

Workflow in NGS

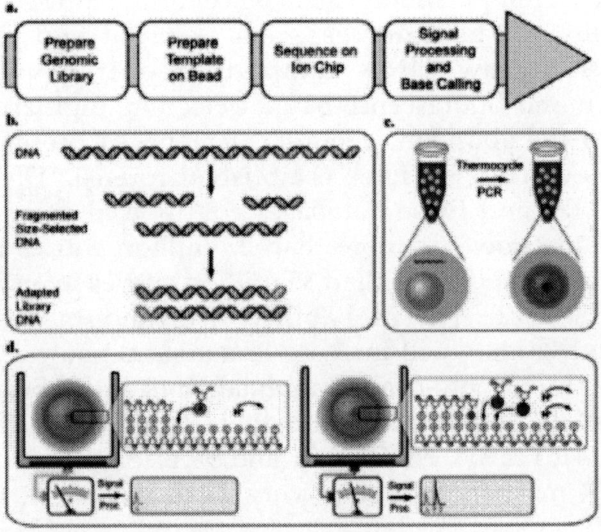

Applications of NGS technology in Wildlife Forensics

The application of DNA technologies in forensic investigations has rendered DNA analysis an important tool in forensic science. Compared to other fields of life sciences, forensic DNA analysis is confronted with template of low copy number, highly-degraded and contaminated samples, the need for high accuracy and reproducibility, as well as time and cost considerations. Today, the majority of forensic DNA tests employ PCR and capillary electrophoresis based fragment analysis methods to detect length variation in short tandem repeat (STR) markers. The CE-based Sanger sequencing has been used to analyze specific regions of mitochondrial DNA (mtDNA) (Jadav *et al.*, 2014). The development of miniaturized gel electrophoresis and the automation of reaction gel loading and signal detection allowed the Sanger methodology to become the gold standard for DNA sequencing. However, CE-based analysis has its limitations, for example, the inability to analyze multiple genetic polymorphisms in a single reaction using a single workflow, low-resolution genotyping of current markers, loss of useful genomic information from degraded DNA samples, and low resolution mtDNA and mixture analysis. These limitations of first-generation sequencing prompt the forensic scientists worldwide to explore the usefulness of NGS technology for forensic studies.

Simple Tandem Repeat (STR) analysis

STR analysis is likely to remain the most important and commonly-used genetic technique in forensic science for the foreseeable future. It displays multiple advantages, such as rapid and precise allele determination, low DNA template requirement, multiplex amplification and fluorescence-based detection, digitized results and utilization of the abundant genomic element, At present, more than 60 countries worldwide have established forensic DNA databases based on STRs, and these databases continue to grow rapidly. For example, China now has more than 27 million entries in its human forensic database and more than 15 million entries in animal forensics (Wang *et al.*, 2012). The probability of a random match between unrelated individuals will increase if statistical analyses were based only on the 13 routinely-used Combined DNA Index System (CODIS) STR markers (*i.e.*, Pati15, Pati18, Pati09, Pati01, 6Hdz700, F124, F53, Fca304, Fca441, Fca954, F85, Fca651 and SRY). Simultaneous detection of more STR markers would be very difficult, due to the technical limitations of fluorescent-based CE sequencers currently in use. Traditional CE-based STR typing using CE is based on the detection of DNA fragment size. Therefore, alleles of identical or similar length but of different sequences cannot be distinguished. Consequently, STR mutations in complex paternity cases often cannot be resolved with traditional CE-based STR analysis. An additional challenge for forensic DNA tests is the analysis of complex DNA mixtures comprising DNA from more than one individual. Contemporary analyses of mixed DNA samples often yield low detection rates, thus are not useful in crime investigations. When NGS technology was firstly introduced to genomics, it was not suitable for STR testing because the read length was generally too short. With technological advances, the average read length has been continually increasing. Since alleles with similar length can be easily distinguished using NGS technology and digital read count could significantly facilitate the identification of mixed DNA samples and analysis of complex paternity cases, some researchers have recently started using NGS technology for STR testing. For example, a pioneer study was performed by Zajac and colleagues, who analyzed three CODIS STR loci, TPOX, CSF1PO and D18S51, using the trinucleotide threading (TnT) approach by 454 Genome Sequencing System (Margulies *et al.*, 2005; Zajac *et al.*, 2009). Subsequently, Irwin *et al.*, 2011 analyzed 13 CODIS STR loci using the 454 GS Junior system in combination with multiplex identifier technology for single source samples. Bornman *et al.*, 2012, went further to show that high-throughput sequencing technology can accurately identify the 13 CODIS STR loci as well as the AMEL gene for not only single source but also mixed samples. To process the forensic NGS data, Warshauer *et al.*, 2013 developed STRait Razor, a software that can analyze the NGS data for 44 STRs, including 23 autosomal and 21 Y chromosome STRs. In addition, Van Neste *et al.*, 2014, used Illumina's MiSeq system to establish a reference allele database to detect single source and mixed DNA samples; they observed that most locus genotyping results were stable and reliable. NGS technology has many potential advantages for STR analysis. These include high throughput, low cost, simultaneous detection of large numbers of STR loci on both autosomes and sex chromosomes, and the ability to distinguish alleles with similar length or digital read count. NGS technology would, therefore, significantly facilitate the identification of mixed DNA samples and analysis of complex paternity cases, and ultimately greatly increase the efficiency and cost-effectiveness of legal cases.

Mitochondrial genome analysis

mtDNA has proved to be a useful forensic tool in cases involving low amounts of DNA or wherein the maternal lineage needs to be investigated, due to its characteristics of small size, multiple copies, maternal inheritance, high mutation rate and lack of recombination. Currently, forensic mtDNA analyses usually detect only polymorphisms within a hypervariable region. However, for mtDNA to be used as a genetic haplotype marker, additional polymorphic loci are required to increase the discrimination power of identification. Therefore, NGS technology has the potential to greatly assist in the analysis of whole mitochondrial sequences. With the increased application of NGS technology in various fields, the cost of equipment and reagents has decreased markedly. Parallel sequencing technology, which allows for simultaneous analysis of multiple samples, has also led to cost-effectiveness. For instance, the number of picotiter plates used in the GS-FLX instrument has increased from 2 to 16, and each channel can simultaneously analyze 192 samples using multiplex identifier (MID) technology. Furthermore, Binladen *et al.*, 2007, used a primer coding technique and produced 256 tagged primers for use in multiple parallel sequencing, allowing 256 samples to be sequenced in a single run. Moreover, Gunnarsdottir *et al.*, 2011, used NGS technology to sequence whole mitochondrial genomes of 109 Filipino individuals at the same time and obtained on average of 55X coverage per sequence, with <1% missing data per sequence. Human mtDNA heteroplasmy is common and heteroplasmy of cells from different tissues within a single individual has also been observed (Cao *et al.*, 2006). mtDNA heteroplasmy is one of the factors affecting the performance of forensic mitochondrial analysis. The detection of heteroplasmy at the whole mitochondrial genome level has been reported (Li *et al.*, 2010), supporting the advantages of using NGS to detect mitochondrial heteroplasmy, including high accuracy and sensitivity, high throughput, low cost, and simple operation (Tang and Huang, 2010). The results of 64 whole mitochondrial genome sequences showed differences in <0.02 % of nucleotides using these two methods and that approximately two-thirds of the differences were observed in or around homopolymeric stretches, since these areas were prone to sequencing errors (Parson *et al.*, 2013).

Phylogenetic analysis of whole mitogenome of Indian domestic pig derived by NGS (Ajit *et al.*, 2016).

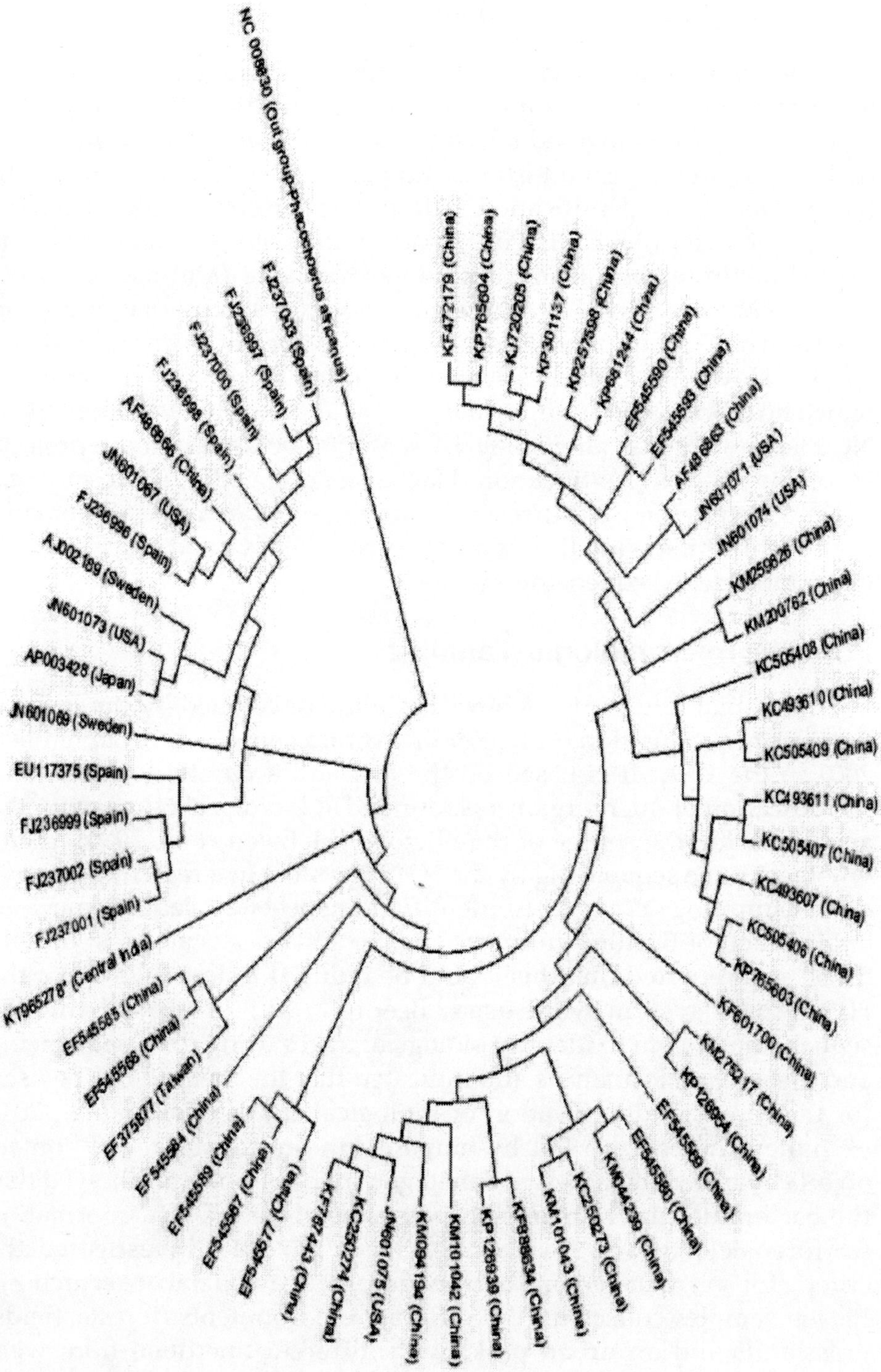
NC 008830 (Out group-Phacochoerus africanus)
KF472179 (China)
KP765604 (China)
KJ720205 (China)
KP301137 (China)
KP257598 (China)
KP681244 (China)
EF545590 (China)
EF545593 (China)
AF486863 (China)
JN601071 (USA)
JN601074 (USA)
KM259826 (China)
KM200762 (China)
KC505408 (China)
KC493610 (China)
KC505409 (China)
KC493611 (China)
KC505407 (China)
KC493607 (China)
KC505406 (China)
KP765603 (China)
KF601700 (China)
KM275217 (China)
KP128964 (China)
EF545569 (China)
EF545580 (China)
KM044239 (China)
KC250273 (China)
KM101043 (China)
KF888634 (China)
KP128939 (China)
KM101042 (China)
KM094194 (China)
JN601075 (USA)
KC250274 (China)
KF787443 (China)
EF545577 (China)
EF545587 (China)
EF545589 (China)
EF545584 (China)
EF375877 (Taiwan)
EF545566 (China)
EF545585 (China)
KT965278* (Central India)
FJ237001 (Spain)
FJ237002 (Spain)
FJ236999 (Spain)
EU117375 (Spain)
JN601069 (Sweden)
AP003428 (Japan)
JN601073 (USA)
AJ002189 (Sweden)
FJ236996 (Spain)
JN601067 (USA)
AF486866 (China)
FJ236998 (Spain)
FJ237000 (Spain)
FJ236997 (Spain)
FJ237003 (Spain)

Animal and plant DNA analysis

Species identification is one of most important components of forensic practice. For example, in cases of poaching (An *et al.*, 2007) and trading of endangered species (Eurlings *et al.*, 2013), it has been used to provide important information and assist in investigations. In the food industry, identification of the species present in meat products can be achieved (Ali *et al.*, 2012), and in archeology, human remains can be distinguished from non-human remains (Malmstrom *et al.*, 2005). At present, most DNA typing methods for species determination are based on PCR amplification using species-specific primers for single species. However, forensic scientists are often faced with situations in which no a priori species information is available. The development of NGS technology has allowed DNA typing to be used in more projects involving species identification (Hajibabaei *et al.*, 2011; Hancock *et al.*, 2013). Cheng *et al.*, 2014, recently identified plants and animals in traditional Chinese medicines using a cost-effective and efficient next-generation deep sequencing method.

Forensic microbiological analysis

Microbial forensics is a new discipline developed by the Federal Bureau of Investigation (FBI) after the Anthrax attack on 18 September, 2001 in the USA. It is based on the fast and accurate detection and identification of microorganisms founded at biological crime, with the aim of tracing the source of the microbe (McEwen *et al.*, 2006). Using whole-genome sequencing by the SOLiD system in a real investigative case, Cummings *et al.*, 2010 identified suspects by sequencing four strains each of Bacillus anthracis and Yersinia pestis at a cost of only $1000 and reported that this would be reduced to less than $50 if the HiSeq 2000 system were used. Brenig *et al.*, 2010 used the 454 sequencing system to identify biological traces using deep sequencing and metagenomic analysis and indicated that the method can be used for the forensic identification of biological traces. Fierer *et al.*, 2010 examined the bacteria left by human skin on the surface of contact objects by using an NGS-based metagenomic method and showed that the bacteria left by human skin possess sufficient DNA information for forensic analysis. A study by Lilje *et al.*, 2013, investigated the criteria for soil metagenome data management and database searching. Eleven samples collected from different environments (forests, fields, grasslands and an urban park) with different microbial flora were sequenced using the Roche/454 platform. The results demonstrated that 18S rRNA gene marker analysis could be used to create and run a filtered database, which was very computationally efficient and flexible. Similarly, Giampaoli *et al.*, 2014 successfully applied a metabarcoding approach to forensic and environmental soil samples, allowing accurate and sensitive analysis of the DNA of microflora, plants, metazoa and protozoa. All the studies described above demonstrate that NGS has the advantages of high throughput, multiplexing capability and accuracy, which makes it suitable for rapid whole-genome typing of microbial pathogens during forensic or epidemiological investigation.

Conclusion

Next-generation sequencing (NGS) is "now generation" and is transforming the capabilities of forensic laboratories. Massively parallel sequencing (MPS) systems enable simultaneous analysis of forensically relevant genetic markers to improve efficiency, capacity, and resolution, bringing modern science in place of outmoded DNA fingerprinting. Advantages of NGS provide the forensic DNA community a revolutionary tool for aiding investigations, including increased information potential, scalability and allelic resolution. Developmental validation data from a targeted forensic NGS system have met forensic DNA quality assurance guidelines with robust, reliable, and reproducible performance on samples of various quantities and qualities (Jager *et al.*, 2017). Although NGS technology appears to have an important role in future wildlife forensic studies, more work is required to fully achieve this goal, which includes overcoming problems with low-template library preparation, error rate, type estimations and issues with NGS data processing and mining.

References

1. Ajit, P.S., Kajal, K.J., Dharmendra, K., Nidhi, R., Awadh, B.S., Bikash, C.S. (2016) Complete mitochondrial genome sequencing of central Indian domestic pig. Journal of Mitochondrial DNA (Part B) Resources, **1:** 949-950.

2. Ali ME, Hashim U, Kashif M, Mustafa S, Che Man YB, Abd Hamid SB. (2012) Development of swine-specific DNA markers for biosensor-based halal authentication. *Journal of Genetics and Molecular Research*, **11**: 1762–72.

3. An J, Lee MY, Min MS, Lee MH, Lee H. (2007) A molecular genetic approach for species identification of mammals and sex determination of birds in a forensic case of poaching from South Korea. *Journal of Forensic Science International*, **167**: 59–61.

4. Berglund, E.C., Kiialainen, A., Syva¨nen, C. (2011) Next-generation sequencing technologies and applications for human genetic history and forensics. *Journal of Investigative Genetics*, **2**: 23-37.

5. Binladen J, Gilbert MT, Bollback JP, Panitz F, Bendixen C, Nielsen R, (2007). The use of coded PCR primers enables highthroughput sequencing of multiple homolog amplification products by 454 parallel sequencing. *Journal of PLoS One*, **2**: e197.

6. Bornman DM, Hester ME, Schuetter JM, Kasoji MD, Minard-Smith A, Barden CA. (2012) Short-read, high-throughput sequencing technology for STR genotyping. *Journal of Biotechniques*, **57**: 1–6.

7. Børsting, C., and Morling, N. (2015) Next generation sequencing and its applications in forensic genetics. *Journal of Forensic Science International and Genetics*, **18**: 78-89.

8. Brenig B, Beck J and Schutz E. (2010) Shotgun metagenomics of biological stains using ultra-deep DNA sequencing. *Journal of Forensic Science International: Genetics*, **4**: 228–31.

9. Budowle, B., Connell, N.D. and Bielecka-Oder, A. (2014) Validation of high throughput sequencing and microbial forensics applications. *Journal of Investigative Genetics*, **5**: 9.

10. Cao, Y., Wan, L.H., Gu, L.G., Huang, Y.X., Xiu, C.X., Hu, S.H. (2006). Heteroplasmy in human mtDNA control region. *Journal of forensic science*, **22**: 190–2.

11. Caratti, S., Turrina, S., Ferrian, M., Cosentino, E., De Leo, D. (2015) MiSeq FGx sequencing system: a new platform for forensic genetics. *Journal of Forensic Science International and Genetics*, **5**: e98–e100.

12. Cheng, X., Chen, X., Su, X., Zhao, H., Han, M., Bo, C., (2014). DNA extraction protocol for biological ingredient analysis of Liuwei Dihuang Wan. *Journal of Genomics Proteomics and Bioinformatics*,**12**: 137–43.

13. Cummings, C.A., Bormann, Chung, C.A., Fang, R., Barker, M., Brzoska, P., Williamson, P.C. (2010) Accurate, rapid and high-throughput detection of strain-specific polymorphisms in Bacillus anthracis and Yersinia pestis by next-generation sequencing. *Journal of Investigative Genetics*, **1**: 5.

14. Eurlings, M.C., Lens, F., Pakusza, C., Peelen, T., Wieringa, J.J., Gravendeel, B. (2013) Forensic identification of Indian snakeroot (Rauvolfia serpentina Benth. ex Kurz) using DNA barcoding. *Journal of Forensic Science*, **58**: 822–30.

15. Fierer, N., Lauber, C.L., Zhou, N., McDonald, D., Costello, E.K., Knight, R. (2010) Forensic identification using skin bacterial communities. *Journal of Protocol of National Acadamy of Science*, **107**: 6477–81.

16. Fullwood, M.J. , C.L. Wei, E.T. Liu, Y. R. (2009) Next-generation DNA sequencing of paired-end tags (PET) for transcriptome and genome analyses. *Journal of Genome Research*, **19**: 521–532

17. Gettings, K.B., Aponte, R.A., Kiesler, K.M., Vallone, P.M. (2015) The next dimension in STR sequencing: polymorphisms in flanking regions and their allelic associations. *Journal of Forensic Science International and Genetics*, **5**: e121-e123

18. Giampaoli, S., Berti, A., Di, Maggio, R.M., Pilli, E., Valentini, A., Valeriani, F. (2014) The environmental biological signature: NGS profiling for forensic comparison of soils. *Journal of Forensic Science International and Genetics*, **240**: 41–47.

19. Gunnarsdottir, E. D., Li, M., Bauchet, M., Finstermeier, K., Stoneking, M. (2011) High-throughput sequencing of complete human mtDNA genomes from the Philippines. *Journal of Genome Research*, **21**: 1–11.

20. Hajibabaei, M., Shokralla, S., Zhou, X., Singer, G.A., Baird, D.J. (2011) Environmental barcoding: a next-generation sequencing approach for biomonitoring applications using river benthos. *Journal of PLoS One*, **6**: e17497.

21. Hancock-Hanser, B.L., Frey, A., Leslie, M.S., Dutton, P.H., Archer, F.I., Morin, P.A. (2013) Targeted multiplex next-generation sequencing: advances in techniques of mitochondrial and nuclear DNA sequencing for population genomics. *Journal of Molecular Ecology Resources*, **13**: 254–68.

22. Hussing, C., Kampmann, M.L., Mogensen, H.S. , Børsting, C., Morling, N.(2015) Comparison of techniques for quantification of next-generation sequencing libraries. *Journal of Forensic Science International and Genetics*, **5:** e276-e278

23. Irwin, J., Just, R., Scheible, M., Loreille, O. (2011) Assessing the potential of next generation sequencing technologies for missing

persons identification efforts. *Journal of Forensic Science International and Genetics,* **3**: 447–8.

24. Jäger, A. C., Michelle, L. A., Carey, P. D., Ernesto, G., Yonmee, H., Lisa, W., Paulina, W., David, S., Nguyen, P., Glorianna, C., Jocelyne, B., Felix, S., Stephanie J., Pond, K., Joe, V., Kathryn, M., Stephens, C., Holt, L. (2017) Developmental Validation of the MiSeq FGx Forensic Genomics System for Targeted Next Generation Sequencing in Forensic DNA Casework and Database Laboratories. *Journal of Forensic Science International and Genetics*, **28**: 52-70.

25. Kajal, J., Nidhi, R., Shrivastav, A.B., Sanju, M., Gaurav, S. (2014) Application of 12S rRNA gene sequence for identification of Indian wild pig (*Sus scrofa cristatus*) . *Journal of Meat Science and Technology,* **2**: 79-84.

26. Kawahara, Y., De la Bastide, M. and Hamilton, J.P. (2013) Improvement of the Oryza sativa Nipponbare reference genome using next generation sequence and optical map data. *Journal of Rice,* **6**: 4.

27. Kothari, N., Schell, M.J. and Teer, J.K. (2014) Comparison of KRAS mutation analysis of colorectal cancer samples by standard testing and next-generation sequencing. *Journal of Clinical Pathology,* **67**: 764-767.

28. Li M, Schonberg A, Schaefer M, Schroeder R, Nasidze I, Stoneking M. (2010) Detecting heteroplasmy from high-throughput sequencing of complete human mitochondrial DNA genomes. *American Journal of Human Genetics,* **87**: 237–4.

29. Lilje L, Lillsaar T, Ra¨ tsep R, Simm J, Aaspo˜ llu A. (2013) Soil sample metagenome NGS data management for forensic investigation. *Journal of Forensic Science International and Genetics,* **4**: e35–6.

30. Malmstrom H, Stora J, Dalen L, Holmlund G, Gotherstrom A. (2005) Extensive human DNA contamination in extracts from ancient dog bones and teeth. *Journal of Molecular Biology and Evolution,* **22**: 2040–47.

31. Margulies, M., Michael, E., William, E.A., Said, A., Joel, Bader, S., Lisa, A.B., Jan, B., Michael, S.B., Yi-Ju, C., Zhoutao, C., Scott, B.D., Lei, D., Joseph, M.F., Xavier, V.G., Brian, C.G., Wen, H., Scott, H., Chun, H. H., Gerard, P. I., Szilveszter, C.J., Maria, L.I.A., Thomas, P.J., Kshama, B.J., Jong-Bum, K., James, R.K., Janna, R.L., John, H.L., Steven, M.L., Ming, L., Jing, L., Kenton, L.L., Hong, L., Vinod, B.M., Keith, E.M., Michael, P.M., Eugene, W.M., Elizabeth, N., John,

R.N., Ramona, P., Bernard, P.P., Michael, T.R., George, T. R., Gary, J.S., Jan, F. S., John, W.S., Maithreyan, S., Karrie, R.T., Alexander, T., Kari, A.V., Greg, A.V., Shally, H.W., Yong, W., Michael, P.W., Pengguang, Y., Richard, F.B. and Jonathan, M.R. (2005) Genome sequencing in microfabricated high-density picolitre reactors. *Journal of Nature,* **437:** 376-380.

32. McEwen, S.A., Wilson,T.M., Ashford, D.A., Heegaard, E. D., Kuiken, T., Kournikakis, B. (2006) Microbial forensics for natural and intentional incidents of infectious disease involving animals. *Review in Science and Technology, Office of International Epizootics,* **25**: 329-339.

33. Oostdik, K., Lenz, J., and Nye, K. (2014) Developmental validation of the PowerPlex® Fusion System for analysis of casework and reference samples: A 24-locus multiplex for new database standards. *Journal of Forensic Science International and Genetics,* **12**: 69-76.

34. Parson W, Strobl C, Huber G, Zimmermann B, Gomes S.M. and Souto L (2013) Evaluation of next generation mtGenome sequencing using the Ion Torrent Personal Genome Machine (PGM). *Journal of Forensic Science International and Genetics,* **7**: 543–49.

35. Pihlstrøm, L., Rengmark, A., Bjornara, K.A.,Toft, M. (2014) Effective variant detection by targeted deep sequencing of DNA pools: an example from Parkinson's disease. *Journal of Annals of Human Genetics,* **78:** 243-252.

36. Sanger,F., Nicklen, S., Coulson, A.R. (1977) DNA sequencing with chain-terminating inhibitors. *Journal of Protocol of National Acadamy of Science,* **74**: 5463–5467.

37. Tang S and Huang T. (2010) Characterization of mitochondrial DNA heteroplasmy using a parallel sequencing system. *Journal of Biotechniques,* **48**: 287–96.

38. Van Neste C, Vandewoestyne M, Van Criekinge W, Deforce D, Van Nieuwerburgh F. (2014) My-Forensic-Loci-queries (MyFLq) framework for analysis of forensic STR data generated by massive parallel sequencing. *Journal of Forensic Science International and Genetics,* **9**: 1–8.

39. Van, D.E.L., Auger, H. and Jaszczyszyn, Y. (2014) Ten years of next-generation sequencing technology. *Journal of Trends in Genetics,* **30**: 418-426.

40. Wang, C., Fullwood, T.E., Wang, T., Wei, E.T. (2012) Application of NGS in forensics. *Proceedings of the 4th International Symposium on New Advances in Forensic Genetics in 2012 (December 9–12) at Fuzhou, China.*

41. Wang, D.Y., Gopinath, S., and Lagacé, R.E. (2015) Developmental validation of the GlobalFiler® Express PCR Amplification Kit: A 6-dye multiplex assay for the direct amplification of reference samples. *Journal of Forensic Science International and Genetics,* **19**: 148-155.

42. Warshauer, D.H., Lin, D., Hari, K., Jain, R., Davis, C., LaRue, B. (2013) STRait Razor: a length-based forensic STR allele-calling tool for use with second generation sequencing data. *Journal of Forensic Science International and Genetics,* **7**: 409–17.

43. Zajac, P., Oberg, C., Ahmadian, A. (2009) Analysis of short tandem repeats by parallel DNA threading. *Journal of PLoS One,* **4**: e7823.

44. Zascavage, R.R., Shewale, S.J., Planz, J.V. (2013) Deep sequencing technologies and potential applications in forensic DNA testing. *Journal of Forensic Science Review,* **25**: 79-105.

□□□